The Great American
Stomach Book

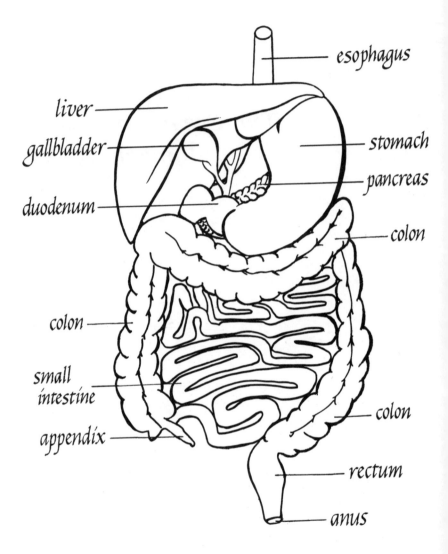

esophagus

liver

gallbladder

stomach

pancreas

duodenum

colon

colon

small
intestine

colon

appendix

rectum

anus

A Simplified View of the Digestive Tract

THE GREAT AMERICAN

Stomach
Book

MAUREEN MYLANDER

Foreword by
HOWARD M. SPIRO, M.D.

Ticknor & Fields
New Haven and New York
1982

Library of Congress Cataloging in Publication Data

Mylander, Maureen.
    The great American stomach book.

    Includes index.
    1. Gastroenterology — Popular works.   I. Title.
RC806.M94   616.3   82-3238
ISBN 0-89919-092-8   AACR2
ISBN 0-89919-108-8 (pbk.)

Diagram on page ii by John O. C. McCrillis

Printed in the United States of America

Q 10 9 8 7 6 5 4 3 2 1

Contents

For Lou, with love

Foreword

by Howard M. Spiro, M.D.
PROFESSOR OF INTERNAL MEDICINE
YALE UNIVERSITY

MOST PEOPLE nowadays want to know everything they can about their bodies so they can take care of minor complaints without going to a doctor. This is as it should be, given the ever-rising cost of medical care and the growth of the self-care movement. Indeed, I like to deal with patients who ask intelligent questions about diagnostic and therapeutic approaches, and about alternatives. I really don't mind — too much — if they question my advice, as long as they know what they are talking about.

Two decades ago, I made rounds with a well-known British gastroenterologist in a leading London hospital. As he passed ceremoniously from bed to bed, he nodded at one patient, "Well, we are going to take away your stomach tomorrow." To which the reply was a grateful, "Oh, thank you doctor!" We have come a long way in two decades. In the United States today that scene would never be repeated because American patients are independent and knowledgeable, and they ask questions. Indeed, the courts have held that the doctor *must* supply information on possible alternative approaches to diagnosis and therapy if the patient is to choose freely and in an informed manner.

That is why this book is so important. Not only does Ms. Mylander tell her readers much about gut disorders, but she takes them through the diagnostic process, even listing some treatments to try out before going to the doctor. She describes the alternatives to the usual approaches that the physician will take, and she discusses the diseases that the physician — and the patient — must consider.

Moreover, she intersperses this with all sorts of good anecdotes and curious facts — from Donleavy, Spallanzani, *The Whole Earth Catalog* — for cocktail party discussion, certainly among gastroenterologists. I learned that a man named Lotito ate a bicycle in fifteen days! I was fascinated to find that Kellogg of cereal fame made an enema machine that could "shoot gallons of water through the bowels in minutes" and that, like the old Viennese physicians, for constipation he prescribed ten to fourteen pounds of grapes a day. Voltaire took enemas for depression, and Kant thought that laughter benefited the gut. There is much more to read and enjoy.

Of course, I do not agree with all that Ms. Mylander has put together. A few general comments in that regard. Maybe Ms. Mylander accepts a little too wholeheartedly the possible connection between diet and physical disorders, but at least she keeps the reader abreast of handouts from the local health food stores along with the latest theories. Dietary therapy has always been important to medical practice, but sometimes it has been more sacramental than physiological. Prescribing diets usually brings out the priest in the physician even if he or she has heard that "Nothing that enters into a man defiles a man." "You are what you eat" meant the most to primitive tribes whose new leader had to eat a part of his predecessor, but today more of us believe that "It is not what you eat, but what eats you" that influences the course of disease.

Still, high-fiber diets have their place and, indeed, are as popular among physicians as among the laity. It is curious, however, that physicians today prescribe the amount of fiber in the diet as punctiliously as they specified the degree of blandness a few years ago. Spinach has a far finer image today than when I was a boy: then it stood for the authority of parents and divided the generations. Now, fathers and mothers on a high-fiber diet to prevent diverticular disease and colon cancer — and incidentally, to scrub their coronary arteries — can greet their doctrinaire and vegetarian children in one great, if sometimes gassy, festival of love. But read what Ms. Mylander has to say and form your own opinions.

She comes out against milk for dyspepsia. To be sure, many gastroenterologists, reading that milk raises the level of gastric acid and believing that acid causes pain, also interdict milk nowadays. Yet so many people have taken it with such good symptomatic results for so long that I think that we have to be careful of too much science and not enough listening. I still prescribe milk for heartburn and indigestion because my patients tell me it is so comforting. Milk may well raise gastric acid levels, but milk is also a fine source of *endorphins* and *exorphins* — substances that relieve pain, among other things. For example, if you mix milk with the proportion of acid and pepsin found in the stomach, the protein in milk is digested into amino acids and peptides, small fragments that turn out to have endorphin activity. It may well be that milk makes the stomach feel better and relieves dyspepsia because it stimulates the flow of those surprising endorphin hormones. The old Greeks may have been right, after all, in talking about the "humors." Now that we know that cholecystokinin and other hormones are found in the brain as well as in the stomach, it may well turn out that the gut influences the brain almost as much as the brain influences the bowel, and that constipation really does lead to headaches!

All in all, I am delighted with what Ms. Mylander tells, though I still suggest milk for indigestion even as I advise plenty of fruits and vegetables and whole grains for constipation. She has given the reader an authoritative layman's view of the digestive tract, managing to keep a balance between the notion that emotion is all-powerful and the faith that what you eat is all that counts.

I will recommend this book to my patients with digestive troubles in the belief that if they read it before they come to see me, they will ask intelligent questions based on what they have read. I may tell them that I disagree with this or that, but I am sure that the person who reads *The Great*

American Stomach Book will be a well-informed patient, maybe even well enough informed to follow his doctor's advice! This is indeed the book that might have been called "Everything You Wanted to Know About Your Stomach, But Didn't Have the Guts to Ask."

Preface

WE LIVE in an age in which people are increasingly attuned to their bodies and what goes wrong with them, and are willing to take responsibility for making themselves well again. These individuals, once dismissed as "health nuts," are gaining in knowledge, credibility, and numbers. They know about their hearts, lungs, brains, and reproductive systems. They understand the microscopic world of the cell, and are even aware of the relationships between mind and body that cause and prolong illness. As Woody Allen said in the film *Manhattan*, "I never get angry; I just grow a tumor!"

Yet, in the midst of this new consciousness, the digestive tract is still terra incognita, and the stomach, liver, gallbladder, pancreas, and intestines remain subject to superstition, ignorance, and taboo. Compared with other major diseases, there is relatively little information available about digestive problems. A few books cover the serious digestive diseases, as this one does, but none are written, as this one is, for those of you who don't have ulcers or liver disease, but who want to know what causes diarrhea, belching, gas, swimmer's cramps, and constipation.

The enemy below, in many cases, could be the food you eat, the way you eat it (too much, too fast, too often), or the emotional tensions and anxieties that affect the way you live and eat your meals. Often the enemy is all three.

Taking care of your stomach and other digestive organs can be difficult when you don't recognize the source of attack, or feel too embarrassed to talk about it. The processes and products of digestion represent one of our society's last taboos. Consider this: sex has been out of the closet for years — thanks, in part, to the fact that between the clinical word and the slang for intercourse, there is the socially acceptable term, *to make love*. But in the English lexicon, there is still no comfortable, socially acceptable word for excrement. However, let us not mince words about feces (or faeces, if you want to be elegant), or about any of the body parts and functions having to do with them. In this book I hope to:

♦ Explore with candor this neglected part of your body and, if necessary, to break taboos that might keep you from appreciating the workings of your digestive tract.

♦ Unveil the feelings and attitudes, especially those of which you are least aware, that can make digestion a pleasure or a problem.

♦ Reassure you about the common complaints and curiosities, in chapters titled "What Makes Sammy Run?", "Looking Out for Number Two," and "Gone with the Wind."

♦ Point out the terrible, unspeakable things you do to your stomach, liver, and other digestive parts.

♦ Warn you about serious problems (ulcers and gallbladder and liver disease) that occur north of the navel, and bowel disorders that can invade your lower depths, and tell you how to prevent, recognize, and deal with them.

♦ Describe the special digestive problems of the very young and very old, and tell you what to expect in each case.

♦ Update you on the latest research developments in gastroenterology, the medical specialty that deals with your gut reactions.

♦ Help you talk candidly to your doctor about your gastrointestinal problems, and tell you what to expect if they need professional care.

Many health books gather dust on America's bookshelves because they are technical and dull, and because they tell you more than you really want to know in language you can't understand. This book is different.

Turn to any part of this book, or read it from start to finish and you will find — in straightforward and, I hope, entertaining language — information meant to help you stop worrying, take better care of yourself, and understand the workings of your digestive tract, from mouth to anus.

It is said that an army travels on its stomach and, therefore, must treat it well. In another idiom, the humorist Josh Billings once wrote, "I hav finally kum to the konklusion, that a good reliable sett ov bowels iz wurth more tu a man, than enny quantity ov brains" (Josh Billings, *His Sayings*, 1865).

Acknowledgments

I WISH TO thank Louis Purdey and Clarissa Wittenberg for their loving support and editing skills, and Col. Roberts H. Billingsley and Mal Schechter for inspiration and launching. For the invaluable time they spent reading and commenting upon the manuscript, I wish to thank Dr. Lon R. White, Dr. Sands K. Irani, Dr. John T. Hagenbucher, and Ms. Miriam Ratner of the American Digestive Disease Society. For suggestions and source material, my thanks to Marc Stern, Irving Shapiro, and Billie Mackey of the National Institutes of Health. Finally, I wish to thank Vivian Cash for typing the manuscript quickly and well; my agent, Carl Brandt, for making this project possible in the first place; and my editor, James Raimes, and publisher, Chester Kerr, for seeing it through.

PART I

Look Out Stomach!

CHAPTER 1

Passages

REMEMBER THE film *Fantastic Voyage?* It was a science-fiction journey through the human body. Four Americans were reduced to microscopic size and injected into the bloodstream of a scientist whose life could be saved only by surgery from within. The rescue team survived giant anti-bodies, withstood the bombardments of the pounding heart, performed the delicate surgery, and exited through the scientist's eye, where the survivors were scooped up in a teardrop.

What if the heroes of *Fantastic Voyage* had traveled through the esophagus and stomach and out through the bowels? Yecchhhhhhh, you say? Yours is a typical response in a society that does not appreciate the wonders of the digestive system. The public has marveled as explorers have penetrated the ocean depths, scaled the highest mountains, and reached out into the vast unknowns of outer space. But few people display the same passion to know about this particular inner space, the murky realms of the digestive tract. For centuries, only a handful of scientists have appreciated and pondered its skillful design.

Hippocrates thought digestion consisted of food somehow cooking itself in the stomach's heat — the origin, perhaps, of the Jewish expression, "May your stomach cook well." Galen decided digestion occurred in the stomach, intestine, and liver, until food was finally converted into blood. Next came some Renaissance gentlemen who thought digestion was a process of fermentation that transformed food into a liquid putrescence. Other authors described digestion as a simple mechanical process in which food was ground and crushed by the undulations of the stomach.

The first reasonably accurate discovery about digestion can be ascribed to a buzzard. In the eighteenth century, a Frenchman named René Antoine Ferchault de Réaumur noticed that his pet buzzard had a nasty habit of regurgitating food that it could not digest. His curiosity aroused, Réaumur somehow induced the bird to swallow sponges. When they came back up, they were soaked in juices, which Réaumur reasoned must be from the stomach. The same juices, he discovered, reduced solid meats to ooze. Réaumur trained other birds and mammals to swallow bits of food tied to wires or strings, which he withdrew after a while to see how much they had decomposed.

Next, an Italian abbé named Lazzaro Spallanzani (1729–1799) did similar experiments on fishes, frogs, snakes, cattle, horses, cats, and dogs. He also conducted some daring experiments on himself to confirm that what's true for animals is also true for humans. After assuring himself that he would probably survive the test, he swallowed little linen bags containing food, just to learn how the digestive system works from end to end.

Late in the eighteenth century, scientists knew that digestion was a chemical process accomplished by the action of gastric juice in the stomach. The English physician William Hunter (1718–1783) summarized the state of the art:

> Some physiologists will have it that the stomach is a mill, others, that it is a fermenting vat, others, again, that it is a stew pan; but in my view of the matter, it is neither a mill, a fermenting vat, nor a stew pan, but a stomach, gentleman, a stomach.

In 1824, William Prout discovered that the stomach produces hydrochloric acid, and in 1833, a milestone work appeared — a book titled *Experiments and Observations on the Gastric Juice and the Physiology of Digestion* (Plattsburgh, N.Y.: F.P. Allen, 1833).

The author, an army doctor named William Beaumont, might never have become famous had it not been for John Jacob Astor's scheme to denude all the fur-bearing animals of North America. It was this enterprise that attracted an eighteen-year-old Canadian, Alexis St. Martin, to one of Astor's trading posts in the Michigan territories. One June day in 1822, as St. Martin stood near his entire winter harvest of pelts, he found himself at the wrong end of a musket that was accidentally discharged about three feet away. The wound was dreadful in appearance: a hole in his chest wall about the size of the palm of your hand. Part of his left lung and stomach protruded through the opening. Food mixed with blood and splinters of rib gushed out. Beaumont, the only physician within a radius of three hundred miles, was summoned. He took one look at the wound, cleaned and bandaged it, and predicted, "The man cannot live thirty-six hours." When he found his patient alive, though not well, the next day, Beaumont revised his prognosis.

Recovery was slow and it left St. Martin, ten months later, in a peculiar condition. His stomach's lacerated edges had attached to his abdominal muscles and formed a fistula, or hole. Beaumont invited the debilitated and destitute St. Martin into his own home, where St. Martin remained for almost two years. Only then did Beaumont decide to use St. Martin's fistula, brimming with digestive juices, to conduct some experiments on digestion. Through the fistula in his patient's stomach, Beaumont lowered pieces of food tied to a silk string, withdrawing them at varying intervals to record what had happened to them.

Every day for the next year or so, St. Martin endured meat, potatoes, bread, fruit, and vegetables until, unstrung at last, he ran away to Canada. There he lived four years, married, and had two children. Beaumont tried to track him down, but to no avail.

In 1829, some fur-trapping friends of Beaumont's lured St. Martin back into the grasp of science. For the next two years, Beaumont, string and notebook in hand, dipped and pulled and learned, among other things, that digestive juices appear in the stomach only when food is eaten.

To prevent further absences without leave, Beaumont drafted a legal agreement in which St. Martin swore to "obey, suffer, and comply with all reasonable orders of the said William in relation . . . to the exhibiting and showing of his said stomach and the powers and properties thereto and of the appurtenances and the powers, properties, and situation and state of the contents thereof." One wonders whether St. Martin — or anybody else — possibly could have known what he was agreeing to. However, St. Martin did seem to understand that he, in turn, would receive board, lodging, and spending money.

Agreements notwithstanding, in 1831 St. Martin again took off for Canada, upsetting Beaumont's plans to exhibit him at a scientific meeting in Europe. But soon afterward, Beaumont did induce St. Martin to travel with him to Washington, D.C. and to enroll in the United States Army as a sergeant. Hereafter, if he ran away, he would be a deserter and would be punished accordingly! The experiments resumed without interruption until November 1, 1833, when Beaumont had enough material for his book. Beaumont later tried to coax St. Martin to return, but his efforts were in vain. At long last, the strange collaboration ended.

Automobiles had not yet been invented, so it could not have occurred to Beaumont that he was looking at a natural carburetor, a mixing bowl in which fuel is combined with air or, in this case, enough hydrochloric acid to dissolve a nail. In a sense, your digestive tract — all thirty feet of it — is much like an internal combustion engine which converts food into the energy that keeps you running smoothly. The digestive system is incredibly sophisticated and involves many complex chemical and physiological processes. Yet its mechanics are, at the same time, amazingly simple.

It all begins in your mouth, where the fuel goes in. Your teeth grind up the food into fine, digestible particles, and saliva starts the work of digesting it. This fluid is produced by small glands under your tongue and in the back of your cheeks. You normally secrete a quart of saliva every twenty-four hours. But let the salivary glands stop when you are nervous or worried, or about to give a speech, and you will notice that your mouth is "dry."

Your tongue pushes food into the esophagus, a whitish pink passageway that measures nine to ten inches and is the fuel pipe to your stomach. The seemingly simple act of swallowing food is actually a series of intricate events involving sensory mechanisms in the mouth and the throat, pathways to the parts of the brain that govern feeding, structures that prevent food from entering the windpipe, and the swallowing muscles themselves. The esophagus has muscles that work so well that you can swallow a glass of water while standing on your head. These wavelike involuntary contractions — called peristalsis — also allow opossums to eat while hanging upside down, and giraffes to drink water while their heads are eight feet lower than their stomachs. Most birds have not been blessed with peristalsis, and so must raise their heads up after each mouthful of water to let gravity help them swallow.

At the bottom of the human esophagus is a valve that closes and keeps food and stomach acids from moving back up the esophagus and into the mouth. However, the valve — like the float in your carburetor — does not always work as it should.

The stomach, a J-shaped organ, can stretch to hold two quarts of food. Or it can collapse, when empty, like a deflated balloon. Although the stomach stores food until it is ready to move into the small intestine, very little digestion goes on in the stomach. Its most important job is to prepare the food chemically and mechanically by mixing it with gastric juice.

As soon as you start chewing food — or even smelling it — your stomach responds by pouring forth a substance containing hydrochloric acid and enzymes, the most important of which is pepsin. Pepsin speeds up the chemical reactions between proteins and hydrochloric acid, but the latter must be present in order for pepsin to do its work.

Nobody knows exactly why the stomach produces these gastric juices, but it is known that they can cause a lot of trouble. If they back into the tender tissues of your esophagus, they can cause heartburn. If your stomach loses its normal ability to resist damage from its own juices, it may start "digesting itself" by developing eaten-away areas called ulcers. If too much of this corrosive gastric juice escapes into the next part of the intestine — the duodenum — it can cause ulcers to form there as well.

When everything functions normally, stomach secretions break down the food you swallow, and the stomach's muscles mix it with a vigorous churning motion to a consistent gruel called chyme. When the chyme is chemically ready, the stomach contracts in waves of peristalsis and moves the chyme toward a valve at its base. This is like the carburetor mixing proper amounts of gas and air before sending the mix to the engine. The stomach empties in small and frequent squirts through the pyloric valve, a rosette of muscle that stands guard to what lies beyond.

What lies beyond is the small intestine, the most vital part of your digestive tract, whose main job is to absorb starches, sugars, proteins, and fats from the food you eat. The small intestine, which measures about twenty to twenty-five feet, compared with the large intestine's five feet, is so named because of its diameter. The small intestine measures about 1½ inches or less — compared with the large intestine's three-inch diameter which, when full, can expand to the width of a rolling pin. Grazing animals, whose food supply is difficult to digest, have longer intestines: a cow's may measure up to one hundred feet long, while a meat-eating animal has a far shorter one. The human intestine, which must digest both animal and vegetable matter, falls somewhere in between.

The first ten to eleven inches of the small intestine — known as the duodenum — is where digestion begins in earnest. The *duodenum*, from the Latin word for *twelve*, was so named because its length was originally measured in finger widths rather than inches. As the stomach's contents enter the duodenum, it releases special hormones into the bloodstream. These chemicals carry messages to two organs: the gallbladder, causing it to release stored bile from the liver into the duodenum, and the pancreas, which pumps pancreatic juice into the duodenum. These digestive juices — like spark plugs igniting the gas and air mix — break the chyme into even smaller particles. Because bile and pancreatic juice are highly alkaline, they neutralize the stomach acid, thereby preventing damage to the duodenum. The skillful design features of this part of your body cause bile and pancreatic juice to flow until all gastric juices are rendered harmless. Then the juices stop until the next injection from your body's carburetor.

Your liver produces a pint or more of bile a day. When it is not immediately needed in the duodenum, the bile drains into the gallbladder. The liver does many other things, but without bile, you could not digest so much as a peanut. The horseshoe-shaped duodenum contains millions of glands which supply even more substances that digest specific foods. You produce up to two gallons of digestive juices daily, which approximates the amount of blood in your body.

Up to this point, the digestive process might seem more like a carwashing operation, with acid and alkaline baths. The chyme is in constant motion as the small intestine contracts / relaxes / contracts / relaxes in the rhythmic ecstasies of peristalsis. But food must do more than just move along. It must also enter the bloodstream through the intestinal walls and from there, move into the body's tissues. This process, absorption, takes place mainly in the first half of the small intestine.

Although the small intestine is little more than twenty feet long, its actual absorptive surface is larger than that of a football field because it contains some four million tiny projections called villi. The villi, which line the intestine's inner surface, contain fine hairlike blood vessels that converge into larger vessels and ultimately connect to the liver. That organ — among its many functions — processes the nutrients and converts them into glucose. When the liver later releases glucose back into the bloodstream, it is carried to the rest of the body. Glucose, the body's major fuel, supplies the body with two-thirds of all its energy.

Energy also comes from fatty acids which enter the body through the intestinal villi and collect into tiny lymph vessels. Lymph is the straw-colored fluid that fills the spaces between the cells throughout your body. So the small intestine is the main reason for the existence of the digestive tract. All the rest — esophagus, stomach, and large intestine — you literally can live without.

If the small intestine, which converts food into energy, is the body's combustion chamber, the large intestine, where practically no digestion takes place, is its exhaust system. When chyme leaves the small intestine, only salt, water, some bile products, and indigestible vegetable fiber remain. As the chyme enters the colon (large intestine), it encounters a T-junction. A left turn leads to the cecum, a cul-de-sac from which hangs the appendix. Both are useless to the digestive process. Turn right, however, and the chyme climbs upward to meet literally trillions of bacteria, which set up a fermentation process with gas bubbles forming and popping. The chyme moves along the five-foot length of the colon — but much slower than before — and eventually, as its remaining water content is sucked into the intestinal wall, ends up a shriveled solid mass. Where twelve ounces of chyme have entered, only about four ounces remain.

The rectum — the last five inches of the colon — can expand to the size of a man's foot. It lubricates and stores the fecal remains until they are ready for release by the strongest valve in the digestive system: the anal sphincter. Ironically, the anus receives its strongest signal to open up just as you begin to eat again. This occurs because the rectum is most likely to transmit a signal to the brain that it is full just as your next meal triggers new waves of peristalsis throughout the intestinal tract. In medical circles, this is known as the gastroileal or gastrocolic reflex.

You've heard the saying, "Ten seconds in the mouth, ten minutes in the stomach, and forever on the hips"? Well, the timing is a little off: food stays in the stomach two to five hours, depending on what you've eaten. Tummy timing is one subject few people understand, yet it is often basic to some of the things that go wrong with your digestive tract.

Retrace the digestive tract once again, this time with a steak dinner and french fries, tossed salad, and a gooey chocolate sundae for dessert, all washed down with two glasses of beer, and coffee. You have handed your stomach a typical challenge. Later, when you realize what you have done, you will apologize and offer it an antacid. But it is timing we are concerned with here, not indigestion. Suppose you eat this meal at 6:00 P.M. Saturday. By 10:30 P.M., your stomach is probably empty, although its emptying time depends upon your mood, and not only upon what you eat. By 1:00 A.M., about three hours later, the food has been thoroughly digested and has just left your small intestine. Now the food moves more slowly through the large intestine. By 6:00 P.M. Sunday, the day after you ate the steak dinner, the first installment of waste from that meal is ready to be eliminated. Not until 6:00 P.M. Monday, however — forty-eight hours after you ate your steak dinner — are the last of its remains ready to leave your large bowel.

This, of course, is the timetable for an *average* meal under *average* conditions. Now consider the variations. The length of time that various foods spend in your stomach and intestines depends upon what you eat, how hungry you are, how much you exercise, and how you feel. The average "transit" time from mouth to anus for the average American diet (low-fiber foods like white bread, sugar, dairy products, processed foods, meats, and fats) is two to four days. In contrast, a high-fiber diet (bran, whole-grain breads and cereals, and raw vegetables and fruits) takes only a day and a half to travel through the digestive tract.

The earliest observations on how long various foods stay in the stomach were made by William Beaumont. He noted that oily substances remained in Alexis St. Martin's stomach for relatively long periods of time. Leafy vegetables stayed longer than meats, and starches were most rapidly eliminated. Later studies confirmed that the composition of a meal influences the length of time it remains in the stomach. Fat generally prolongs the process, while a meal composed of pure proteins or starches shortens it. In one recent study of transit times of various foods, it was found that the traditional high-fiber diet of Ugandan villagers — consisting mainly of maize, plantain, and legumes — took about thirty-three hours to pass through the gut, while low-fiber, institutional diets in an English boarding school and the British

Navy took from seventy-six to eighty-three hours — or up to 3½ days — to pass through.

Other investigators have reported that hunger, mild exercise, and cold weather shorten emptying time, while exhausting exercise and hot weather slow it down. This suggests why you might feel more hungry during cold weather — your stomach empties sooner — and less hungry when the temperature soars.

Emotions also influence gastric emptying time. Food served in pleasant surroundings hastens digestion, while food served under emotional stress prolongs the process. Anger, fright, and worry may slow down secretions of digestive juices and make digestion take longer. However, feelings of anxiety and insecurity may speed up the process and cause diarrhea.

Certain substances cause their own unique gut reactions and timings. For example, liquids, especially water taken alone or with food, leave the stomach rapidly and are absorbed into the bloodstream through the intestines within minutes if you are very thirsty. You take in about 1.2 quarts of water daily through liquids, and about a quart through the food you eat. The average person loses 2½ quarts of water daily — about a quart through urine, and smaller amounts through sweating, breathing, and defecating.

Alcohol, by contrast, can be absorbed into the bloodstream directly from the stomach, which is why you can become intoxicated quickly when drinking on an empty stomach. Thus, alcohol can be detected in the blood five minutes after it is swallowed. However, most alcohol, especially the first drink, is absorbed into the bloodstream from the small intestine, which has no control over its rate of absorption. After that, alcohol irritates the stomach lining and decreases its activity so that subsequent drinks remain in the stomach longer and continue to be absorbed directly into the bloodstream from that organ.

Alcohol diluted with water is absorbed rapidly, whereas alcohol taken with milk or other fats takes longer to absorb. The length of time it takes the body to metabolize or get rid of alcohol also depends, in large part, upon what size you are, what kind of alcohol you drink and how fast you drink it. A 160-pound man who drinks one Zombie, a very strong rum drink containing 2.5 ounces of pure alcohol, will take 9.8 hours to metabolize it. The same man will take 2.7 hours to get rid of a highball containing 1.5 ounces of liquor, 2.3 hours to metabolize a glass of table wine, and 1.9 hours to metabolize a beer.

When you swallow a pill, your body similarly tries to use part of the drug and eliminate the rest. Most drugs are absorbed in the small intestine and only a few, most notably alcohol and aspirin, are absorbed in the stomach. Thus, many drugs have an enteric coating that will not dissolve in the acid environment of the stomach and will arrive intact in the duodenum. There, drugs that dissolve in fat enter the bloodstream and go to the liver to be transformed into compounds that can be eliminated in urine.

Timing depends upon the kind of drug you take. Each substance has a half-life, which is the amount of time it takes to eliminate half the drug from your body. This may range from a few minutes to several weeks, and varies from person to person. That is why your doctor may tell you to take a drug for a week or longer, so that it can reach a state of maximum efficiency during which as much drug is absorbed as is eliminated within twenty-four hours.

Other gut reactions, such as vomiting, intestinal gas, or diarrhea, have their own timing. Because these are complex interactions — depending upon what and how much you have eaten, how you feel, what organisms may have invaded your body, and how well your digestive tract is functioning — they will be discussed in later chapters.

Every person has his or her own unique digestive chemistry, but the basic processes are the same. And regardless of individual differences, two factors appear to have an enormous influence on digestion and health: what you put into your stomach and how you feel when you eat or drink it.

These two themes you will hear again and again.

CHAPTER 2

The Toilet Taboo

In November 1979, The American Digestive Disease Society (ADDS), a voluntary health organization, launched a telephone answering service in Washington, D.C. called *Gutline*. Its purpose is to inform the public about digestive diseases and to help people who have them. On two evenings a week, at no cost, callers throughout the country are able to speak to a doctor about personal digestive problems, and to learn whether they need further medical attention. In the first three months of operation, the service attracted hundreds of callers. Although a few were well informed, an ADDS spokesperson said, "The ignorance about digestive diseases is appalling."

In May 1981, the ADDS conducted a test of *Gutline* in New York at a professional meeting of gastroenterologists. In a four-day period, telephone lines manned by four to six doctors, ten hours a day, were swamped by twenty-two hundred phone calls from all over the country. Again, some of the callers were well informed about their diseases, but most were miserable and essentially uninformed about what was happening to them. "In other words, the national experience," the ADDS spokesperson noted, "paralleled what we had found in Washington." (For more information about *Gutline*, see Appendix A.)

14

The National Commission on Digestive Diseases — which was commissioned by Congress in 1976 to study digestive diseases in the United States — had reported in 1979 that twenty million Americans suffer constantly from severe digestive diseases, and fourteen million more suffer occasionally from these same disorders. For two years, in city after city, the Commission collected personal accounts of affliction with digestive diseases. When all the stories were told and transcribed, the catalog of suffering weighed four hundred pounds. The Commission concluded that digestive disorders, despite their toll, are perhaps the least studied and least understood of all ailments that plague mankind. The final report suggested why: "The digestive tract and its functions are viewed through veils of ignorance, embarrassment, taboo, and inappropriate humor."

All of us have learned, one way or another, to observe the "toilet taboo." At the age of two, I swallowed a 1911 Liberty nickel. My parents watched anxiously for it to reappear. Two days. Five days. A week. They took turns checking my chamber pot until, two weeks later, on a bleary-eyed New Year's Day morning, my mother managed to fish it out.

This story has been told and retold so many times that it has become the foremost anecdote of my childhood. Only recently was I told — because I was writing a book — the even seamier story of an earlier time when I smeared the walls, sides of my screened-in kiddy-coop bed, and myself from head to toe with the solid waste products of my infant body.

After the nickel crisis, bathroom activities receded from consciousness, and I learned to ignore my tummy and its end products. But years later, I wondered how many 1911 Liberty nickels are preserved, as mine is, between the yellowing pages of baby books? And how many fecal wonder stories remain untold between the lines of baby books throughout the land? From the first day your parents decided that you must become "socially acceptable," that is, toilet-trained, the lower end of your anatomy became the terrain over which the battle of the bowel would be waged.

Your parents are not to be condemned for their zeal, for they, in turn, fought the same war with their parents —

and lost. Down through the generations, the terms of surrender have always been the same: henceforth, you will stop defecating at will — a natural instinct — and do so at your parents' will — an unnatural instinct. You will also learn to coordinate some complex neuromuscular actions and, above all, to *strain*.

The United States Government even came to the aid of parents in enforcing this unwritten Eleventh Commandment. In its popular pamphlet *Infant Care*, published in the 1920s, the Children's Bureau stated, "Training of the bowels may be begun as early as the end of the first month. It should always be begun by the third month and may be completed during the eighth month." The pamphlet urged that the time of day for this activity should never vary, not even by five minutes, and offered detailed instructions for inserting a soap stick into the rectums of noncompliant children.

Now the prevailing theory is to wait until at least age fifteen months to *begin* toilet training. Whatever age it begins, however, the message is clear: there is one unwaivable requirement for acceptance into society. It is not that you must have good table manners, or obey the laws, or learn how to read, or refrain from beating your children, deserting your spouse, or taking the life of another person. All of these things — under one circumstance or another — you may do. But if you fail to learn bowel control, you insure banishment from the company of your fellow man. Indeed, fecal incontinence is the main reason that many old people are consigned to nursing homes. An untrained bowel is the one thing society will not tolerate.

It has always been so, although early toilet practices appear to have been governed more by sanitary considerations than by social hang-ups. The Moslems were — and still are — allowed to use only the left hand for cleaning themselves after eliminating; they use the right one for eating. Hindus carried a vessel of water to a secluded area to wash their feet before eliminating, and to wash their anal regions afterward. The Romans built sewers leading to the Tiber, introducing the modern concept of a sewage (though not a sanitary) system. During the Middle Ages, sanitary conditions and consciousness regressed. In Europe, the common people dumped their waste into city streets while the nobility dumped theirs into various smelly moats. Not until the mid-nineteenth century did modern sewers and toilets make their debut.

Enter Thomas Crapper, inventor of the flush toilet, whose name might have passed into obscurity had it not been for American soldiers returning from World War I. They could not erase from their memories of war-torn Europe the Crapper name-brand that appeared on English toilets, and thus introduced his last name, at least, to America.

Crapper's story is told by Wallace Reyburn in *Flushed With Pride: The Story of Thomas Crapper* (London: MacDonald and Company, 1969). Reyburn recounts that Crapper was a Chelsea plumber who went to work at age eleven, and ended up discussing sanitary arrangements with several English monarchs. Although Crapper also may be credited with inventing the stair tread, his most significant contribution was his improvement of the flush toilet, which, before Crapper made his mark on it, sent water gushing from a cistern after the user pulled the chain. The problem was that water flowed endlessly through the bowl because the valves leaked and because people forgot to close them — a waste of water, Crapper thought.

Thus Crapper's offering, the Water Waste Preventer, was shown at the Health Exhibition of 1884 in England. There, according to press reports, it completely cleared away ten apples, four pieces of paper, one flat sponge, and an unrecorded amount of plumber's "smidge" — a challenge even for contemporary toilets. Thomas Crapper, his career secure, was appointed sanitary engineer to His Majesty, Edward VII, and later, to George V. Euphemisms proliferated. Crapper's brainchild became known as the "loo," "biffy," "chamber of commerce," or "shot-tower." When people wanted to use it, they would do everything from "seeing a man about a dog" to going to *"telephoner à Hitler,"* a euphemism used by French Resistance workers during World War II. In Denmark, women — perhaps inspired by the French — asked for the ladies' phone, and in New Zealand, the native Maoris went to the *whare-noho* ("sit-house"). The term "john" — referring to the trade name of the toilet — was dignified in a regulation issued at Harvard University in 1735, stating that "no Freshman shall go into the Fellows 'John'."

In his classic letters to his son, Lord Chesterfield wrote in 1747 of a man who bought a common edition of Horace and gradually tore off the pages, carrying them to the "necessary room." There he read them first, and then "sent them down as a sacrifice to Cloacina," the sewer goddess. In this manner, he worked his way through all the Latin poets.

Toilet paper came along somewhat later. Reyburn listed sixty euphemistic words and phrases for this commodity in his book about Crapper, and said he was just scratching the surface. In Victorian England, for example, shopping housewives called it "curl paper" to avoid the embarrassment of having to ask for toilet paper in the store. At that time, toilet paper came in separate squares that resembled the papers women used to curl their hair. The inventor of the toilet roll is not known, but the product came into widespread use after two Philadelphia brothers named Scott popularized this new advance in Western civilization.

Outhouses — perhaps the ultimate embodiment of the toilet taboo — consigned the bowel to the back yard and beyond. In time, outdoor plumbing moved indoors — you may think, to stay. A new development, however, has occurred with the recent appearance of a catalog titled *Privy: The Classic Outhouse Book* (Delafield, Wisc.: Sun Designs, 1981). It features twenty-five original outhouse plans, including a movable model called the "Prairie Schooner," and others known as the "Roman Bath," "Marblehead," "Olde Bailey," and "Knob Hill." Some are large enough to accommodate woodburning stoves, glass-topped coffee tables, gym equipment, or several easy chairs. Accessories include skylights, weathervanes, and macramé tissue holders. The "Chalet" model features a built-in puppet stage, demonstrating that outhouses have come a long way since the wild, wild West, when some privies had gun ports in case of attack.

The finer qualities of the bathroom have not been lost upon author J.P. Donleavy who, in a book of humorous essays titled *The Unexpurgated Code: A Complete Manual of Survival and Manners* (N.Y.: Delacorte Press, 1975), described the "crapularium" as the place where you spend what should be "the most profound moment of your day." He advises that the crapularium be provided with selected reading material on your favorite subjects. And to insure that the solemnity of those surroundings never be interrupted, even when you are traveling, Donleavy advises always carrying an easily attached *Out of Order* sign.

Now, how to introduce the product of that "most profound moment"? Historically? Throughout the ages, excrement has been a major ingredient in many popular medicines. The medicinal use of these human and animal excretory products is called "coprotherapy."

Archaeologically? The discovery of a "privy pit" or a "coprolite," as fossil-hunters call it, is cause for excitement, for such findings reveal a great deal about man's ancestors. Into privy pits, for example, have been tossed pottery, eating implements, tools, and other household discards, illustrating that one man's trash is another man's treasure. Dessicated human feces found in or near prehistoric camps and dwellings reveal information not only about the diets and seasonal activities of early hunters and farmers, but also about their state of health, techniques of food preparation, and environmental conditions. The analysis takes place in a laboratory. The specimen is immersed in a diluted solution of trisodium phosphate for at least seventy-two hours and — voila! — is revealed to belong to a grass-eating animal (if the fluid remains translucent or yellowish) or to a meat-eating mammal (if it turns pale brown). If, however, the fluid turns opaque and dark brown or black, it belongs either to a human or to a coatimundi, a racoonlike creature that is the only mammal whose feces are known to give a similar reaction. The coprolite is then passed through a twenty-mesh brass screen, followed by a one-hundred–mesh screen. What's left is dried and placed under a microscope, which may reveal bits of charcoal picked up in cooking, plant fibers, seeds, hairs, bone, nutshell, eggshell, feathers, and the hard parts of insects. The greater the variety, the clearer the evidence that the specimen is from a human.

Psychologically? People vary, and what fascinates one repels another. In the psychological sense, matters of the bowel cause more anxiety, and evoke more hidden symbols than perhaps even sex. One need not subscribe to the theories of Sigmund Freud to recognize the common sense in his observation that feces are one of a child's earliest "creations." Like writing a book, they are satisfying to produce, but do not always get good reviews. Timing is one of the keys to success or failure. Produced at the right time and place, the output wins nothing but praise from parents. Produced at the wrong time and place, or used as a plaything, smeared on walls or — worst of all — not produced at all, feces are the child's ultimate *gotcha* to the parents! It is enough to impress indelibly upon all concerned that this body product is a source both of power and of shame. It is also a source of fear: many children think that when they have a bowel movement, they lose a vital body part.

From such powerful wellsprings come many anxieties about the bowel. There is also — and you need not have read the works of Masters and Johnson or Alex Comfort to recognize it — an unspoken connection between elimination and sexual functions. Thus, some people avoid rectal examinations by a physician even when there is obviously something wrong. The toilet taboo takes hold early. One seven-year-old was bleeding from the rectum, but for many weeks would not tell her mother because she was afraid to admit that she even looked at her bowel movements (although nearly everybody does, and should). The overtones of sexuality, even more than the undertones of toilet-training, make the digestive tract — especially its lower end — conversationally taboo.

Imagine, then, the public relations — not to mention the interplanetary health — implications of feces disposal during space voyages. The challenges of synthetic diets, palatability, food preservation, and the like, pale before the question of what to do in weightless outer space when it comes out the other end. Proposals for waste management on extended space flights have ranged from drying fecal matter with heat or dry air to pressure-filtering, incinerating, and processing it into sludge.

But theory outstripped practice in the early days of the space program, particularly during the Mercury III flight in May 1961, when astronaut Alan Shepard prepared to become the first American in space. Nobody had thought to provide a urine receptacle — after all, the flight was to last only fifteen minutes — and nobody anticipated that the countdown might drag on for hours. Finally, as the tide in his bladder became unbearable, Shepard requested — and received — permission to "do it in the suit." The flood partially knocked out his electrocardiogram sensors and perturbed his physicians, but did not cause NASA to scratch the flight. NASA later designed an in-suit system for urinating, consisting of a condom attached to a rubber bag strapped to the hips, and a tight-fitting elastic garment that was, in essence, a diaper. But since astronauts spend relatively little time in their space suits, NASA invented more elaborate fecal containment systems (FCS) for use in the spacecraft.

Rusty Schweickart, the first astronaut to venture outside the space capsule on the Apollo IX mission, described urination and defecation in zero-gravity in an interview with Peter Warshall in *The Next Whole Earth Catalog* (Sausalito, Calif: Point, 1980), published as an article titled "There Ain't No Graceful Way." According to Schweickart:

> . . . In Apollo, for feces you just stuck a plastic bag on your butt. . . . Hopefully centrally located. . . . But then the problem comes, because there's no particular reason whatsoever for the feces to separate from your rear end. . . . From the time you start to peel down to stick the bag on and all that, till the time you have finished cleaning up . . . it's damn near an hour. And at times it's taken longer.

During the Skylab missions, fecal facilities improved. Each man had his own collection system consisting of a seat against which he sealed his rear end while an airflow substituted for gravity and carried the feces into a collection bag.

> SCHWEICKART: . . . the system worked well. But then after you did that, you sort of stuff the bag with wiping paper, seal it, then weigh it to get the mass, the wet mass, and then put it into a vacuum oven to bake. . . . then you'd stick it in the stack with all the other cow pies and bring them all home for analysis. . . .
> WARSHALL: A lot of people were wondering what happens when you start dumping things into space. . . .
> SCHWEICKART: Well, the only thing that (got) dumped into

space is the urine, and that no longer is dumped into space. . . . The fecal matter has always been stored on board.

WARSHALL: Oh, I see. People have visions of fecal matter and urine ruining space.

SCHWEICKART: No, no. The only thing that is left floating around out there is principally water which instantly flashes into ice crystals. . . .

WARSHALL: So somewhere out in space is just some sublimated water crystals floating around.

SCHWEICKART: Yeah.

WARSHALL: Well you can see what they were worried about. Some day the sun's rays . . . blocked out by . . .

SCHWEICKART: It's all stored aboard, so they don't have to worry about it.

Despite the worries they cause, feces also have some positive potential. Nitrogen, methane, and other gases generated by human and animal manure can heat hog pens, houses, and even cook food. In fact, excrement is one of the "Big Five" sources of alternate energy. The grass is greener on many a golf course because it has been fertilized with a spray made from ground human excrement mixed with water. In Asian cultures such as Japan, human excrement — called night soil — has traditionally been used as a fertilizer to raise vegetables. If these crops were eaten raw and unpeeled, they could spread intestinal parasites. Thus, Allied troops occupying Japan after World War II were not allowed to eat crops grown in Japanese soil. Nevertheless, the contamination problem could be solved, despite the regulations, by washing these vegetables in hypochlorite solution (Chlorox). Maj. Gen. Douglas B. Kendrick, who was Gen. Douglas MacArthur's personal physician at the time, tells of an occasion when he gave this advice:

. . . Mrs. MacArthur (in 1946) received the most beautiful box of strawberries I had seen. They were individually placed in a box of cotton like a group of rubies. Mrs. Mac called and said, 'Joe, what do we do with these?' and I said, 'Soak them for thirty minutes in ten parts per million of hypochlorite and they'll be perfectly safe and good.' An hour later Mrs. Mac called and said she was sending the strawberries down to me.

General Kendrick, who was retired and living in Tampa, Florida, at the time of this writing, told me that his conclusion about this incident is: "You must have faith!"

Today, composting toilets are turning human waste into night soil in many parts of the United States, despite resistance from public health and sewage authorities. Composting advocates contend that we should stop putting our bodily wastes in the water, where they don't belong, and put them on the land, where they do belong. Composting toilets, the argument goes, conserve water and, in as little as six months, can break human waste into an odorless, rich, disease-free fertilizer for flowers, fruit trees, and crops such as beans or corn that do not come into direct contact with the soil.

Consider the potential: stools vary in size from four to eight inches long by one to 1½ inches wide. The stools of vegetarians are generally larger, softer, and less odorous than those of meat-eaters. The average human produces a half-pound (moist weight) of feces daily and a quart of urine, or a yearly average of about 180 pounds of feces and ninety gallons of urine. For composting purposes, this is equivalent to less than three cubic feet of feces and about twelve cubic feet of urine before evaporation and decomposition. The urine contains from ten to fifteen percent nitrogen, or ten pounds of pure nitrogen per year. The feces consist of sixty-five percent water, ten to twenty percent ash, ten to twenty percent soluble substances, and five to ten percent nitrogen.

Thus, feces have fascinated infants, frustrated parents, confounded astronauts, and fertilized flowers. And that is not all. Bowel movements also serve as vital indicators of your state of health and provide early warning signals of disease. Yet many people are too embarrassed to tell even their doctors about a function that is — however much they despise, deny, and disclaim it — one of the basics of life and good health.

CHAPTER 3

Gut Reactions

SCENE FROM a recent workshop of the National Foundation for Ileitis and Colitis (NFIC): a gastroenterologist pointed out that many of her patients with inflammatory bowel disease are depressed. Could their depression, she asked, be a cause of their disease? Her colleagues groaned audibly, and one replied, "I'd be depressed too if I were having twenty bowel movements a day!"

The question — a very serious one — deserves a careful answer. Are digestive diseases emotionally induced? Psychiatrists, psychologists, and people who believe that stress can affect your body's reactions and cause disease tend to think so.

Yet many people who suffer from and / or treat digestive diseases think not. A pamphlet published by the NFIC on emotional factors in ileitis and colitis — inflammatory diseases of the small and large bowel — asks, "Can tension and anxiety cause ileitis and ulcerative colitis?" And answers, "In ulcerative colitis, a condition which is associated with inflammation or structural changes, there is no evidence that emotions play a causative role. . . . It is very important to correct this common and erroneous impression."

But among gastroenterologists, the physicians who specialize in digestive diseases, the tide may be turning. The first chapter of a major medical reference text edited by M.H. Sleisenger and J.S. Fordtran titled *Gastrointestinal Disease* (2d. ed., Philadelphia: W.B. Saunders Company, 1978), states that the vast majority of patients' digestive complaints to physicians cannot be linked to a physically recognizable disease or disorder, but rather, indicate abnormal adaptations to life stress. The textbook defines life stress as "any situation regarded by an individual as a threat to his security. The situation may be real, anticipated, or fantasized, for its determining characteristic is its meaning to the person affected."

For years, studies of stress and peptic ulcers have noted that ulcer patients tend to experience more emotional tension and stresses from occupational and financial crises than people without this physical condition. During World War II, repeated air raids in England, Sweden, Switzerland, and Germany created prolonged stress that caused peptic ulcer rates to soar in those countries. Head injuries, major surgical procedures, and severe illnesses can also produce "acute stress ulcers," or multiple erosions in the stomach and duodenum.

The Sleisenger and Fordtran text notes that sometimes stress affects the function of, say, the bowel, without causing any change in its structure. These are called psychophysiologic reactions to general stress. In an introductory section titled "The Gastrointestinal Tract in Man Under Stress," the text adds that patients with inflammatory bowel disease "have been found to be relatively incapable of experiencing or finding words to describe strong emotion." When such patients do begin to express their feelings about their lives and their disease when they first undergo psychotherapy, their physical illness often gets worse abruptly, and then gets better. Another leading textbook, *Gastroenterology*, edited by Abraham Bogoch (N.Y.: McGraw-Hill, 1973), notes that ". . . there seems to be little doubt that emotional conflict plays a major role in most cases of ulcerative colitis. . . ."

One out of every two Americans periodically suffers from a digestive disorder that he does not take to a physician. Since most of the complaints that *are* taken to physicians are emotionally induced, it is probable that many, if not most, of the tummy troubles treated at home have emotional roots as well.

The American Digestive Disease Society (ADDS) also periodically reminds its members of tension's toll on the digestive system. One ADDS publication points out that emotional problems can cause skin trouble, blood pressure problems, and may even cause dental disorders in people who grind their teeth while sleeping. So why not digestive problems as well? "Most of us want to deny that our lifestyles are causing us trouble," the ADDS newsletter adds, "but these problems are all too common, so relax and do something about it." The ADDS advice is to have your physician check you for physical causes. If none are found, ". . . you can start dealing with what is probably the main problem. As in so many 'mind over matter' situations, once you decide to deal with the real problems, you are able to do something about them."

The idea that you express your emotional tensions through your gut is not a new one. Since earliest times, the human digestive tract has expressed man's most pressing needs for survival. When enemies threaten, the mouth goes dry, the stomach shuts down, and the bowels empty in a carry-over of a weight-lightening function — all in preparation for fight or flight.

King George III of England developed a bad case of indigestion whenever he became enraged or frustrated. As news of the Boston Tea Party and the like reached his ears, these attacks became more and more frequent. To soothe his stomach, he would eat a single boiled potato. But the basic cause of his indigestion — his reaction to news of the deteriorating situation in the Colonies — was something he never remedied.

William Beaumont observed that whenever Alexis St. Martin felt angry, his emotions affected the digestion of food in his stomach, including how fast it passed through. St. Martin had cause for anger. After all, Beaumont *had* prevailed upon him to enroll in the United States Army.

Another classic study of gut reactions involved a person named Tom (only his doctors know his last name). In 1895, when Tom was nine, the walls of his esophagus became fused together when he drank scalding-hot clam chowder. He could never swallow again. His doctors fashioned a stoma, or hole, that led directly into his stomach so food could be poured in. Tom chewed it and then spat it into an ordinary kitchen funnel inserted into his stoma. Through this window — similar to the one in Alexis St. Martin's stomach — Drs. Stewart Wolf and Harold L. Wolff of New York Hospital studied Tom's stomach. Drs. Wolf and Wolff, who specialized in physical reactions to stress, befriended Tom and got him a job in the hospital. It became obvious that the lining of Tom's stomach reacted according to his mood. When he felt dejected and overwhelmed by a situation — for example, when he was afraid of losing his job or when he went to see a government official about adopting his stepgrandchildren — his stomach reacted by underfunctioning. He had been eating a breakfast of two eggs scrambled in butter, one slice of buttered bread, a pint of milk, and several cups of weak coffee. Under normal conditions, this breakfast emptied from his stomach in about six hours. But during this period of fear and dejection, emptying time was an hour longer than average, and the lining of his stomach became pale, produced far less acid, and did not contract as vigorously as usual.

By contrast, when Tom felt angry, frustrated, and hostile — for example, when someone criticized his work — his stomach lining turned fiery red and poured forth gastric juices. Stomach contractions increased and his breakfast was emptied in four to five hours, compared to the normal five to six.

His stomach's reactions also mirrored the degree and duration of his emotional reactions. Tom was usually disturbed over financial problems, and was compelled to accept help from a certain benefactor. When the benefactor threatened to withdraw financial support unless allowed to meddle in Tom's personal affairs, Tom became intensely anxious and resentful. This caused a prolonged period of accelerated gastric function: acids poured forth, the stomach membrane became red and enlarged, and Tom suffered from frequent heartburn and abdominal pain. In addition, the lining of his stomach became far more susceptible to injury at such times.

Even stroking it with dry gauze caused bleeding and small erosions. These injuries usually healed in twenty-four hours or less.

Dr. Harold Wolff once described Tom as "not the sort of person who harbors grudges or maintains emotional stress for prolonged periods. Usually he expressed his feelings in words or in action . . ." In later years, however, Tom developed ulcers and cancer. The cancer was successfully removed, but when his doctors tried in 1956 to convince Tom to have surgery for his ulcer, he refused and ended a twenty-year relationship with his two physician friends. He died shortly thereafter.

Subsequent studies have shown that what Drs. Wolf and Wolff observed inside Tom's stomach, happens unseen on a daily basis in everyone's stomach. The degree and duration of the changes, and whether or not they cause harm, depends upon how well you handle stress.

Hans Selye, a noted authority on stress, says that if an alarming or abnormal condition continues for a long time, your ability to adapt to it wears out, and a stage of exhaustion develops during which further resistance becomes impossible. According to this theory, ulcers are an example of an inability to adapt to stress. Stress affects the digestive system in other ways as well. Nausea, for example, often has psychological roots. Studies showing relationships between emotional stress and the intestine are not as numerous as those relating to the stomach. Several studies, however, show that fear and dejection are associated with lack of color and activity of the colon. One soldier was totally constipated for six weeks during jungle fighting behind enemy lines in World War II, an adaptation that may have helped him to survive by protecting him from parasites, detection, and vulnerability to enemy attack.

In a gut reaction triggered by strong feelings, the lining of one medical student's colon reddened as if it were blushing when he discovered — in a situation that was deliberately set up to see how he would react — that the examiner at the other end of a sigmoidoscope that had been inserted into his rectum, was a woman doctor.

And who can deny that lovesickness causes pulses to quicken, tears to form, breath to grow short, and knots to form in the stomach and gut? Emotions can cause — in the lovelorn and loveless alike — a bitter taste in the mouth, burping, intestinal gas, loss of appetite, constipation, diarrhea, ulcers, spastic colon, and hemorrhoids. Later chapters will discuss the role that emotions play in each of these disorders. Some investigators claim that people with certain personality traits tend to develop diseases such as ulcers and inflammatory bowel disease. Many studies show that people who have such diseases tend to be depressed and unable to express their feelings, especially their resentments. Indeed, there is considerable evidence that some people mask feelings of depression and its accompanying sense of helplessness, hopelessness, and haplessness by complaining of physical illness. This is the only way they feel free to express these feelings. In medical circles, this phenomenon is known as "organ language."

The theory that some people have an "ulcer personality" or an "ulcerative colitis personality," however, does not enjoy universal acceptance. Although it recognizes that emotions can play a part in digestive disorders, the American Digestive Disease Society says that the "ulcer personality" is largely a myth, and that few popular beliefs about ulcer-prone people are supported by clinical investigation. The National Foundation for Ileitis and Colitis contends that the concept of an "ulcerative colitis" or "ileitis personality" is not only a myth, but a way of blaming the patient for having the disease.

So the controversy rages on, with few real facts to settle it. Dr. Denis McCarthy, an expert in digestive diseases and ulcers, formerly from the National Institutes of Health, acknowledges that studies about the stress background from which ulcers develop have not been very imaginative. Other investigators note that the nervous system might be overtaxed to the point of developing physical disease, but acknowledge that there is often little inclination to pursue the matter — or the patient's psychological situation — more deeply.

Why are we so reluctant to use psychotherapy and other forms of counseling to explore our own inner space, especially when the digestive tract offers such a visible laboratory for studying the links between body and mind? Could it be that exploring our lower depths and learning about our own particular gut reactions would reveal secrets we keep even from ourselves?

CHAPTER 4

The Way We Eat

I'd just finished a cup of hot chocolate, and Frank brought me a Coke to wash down the peanuts. Then, after eating the two boxes of dried raisins and the package of dried fruit, I was just thinking about having the sardines when . . .

(Office worker recalling his mid-afternoon snack)

OH STOMACH, oh duodenum, oh liver, gallbladder, and bowel: how we abuse you! We pamper our hearts, attend to toothaches, and rush to remedy anything that blemishes our skin. But to our stomach's gentlest pleas for kind treatment, we refuse to give audience.

Moses Maimonides, the twelfth-century physician and philosopher, wrote that digestive troubles stem from eating too much, eating poor-quality food, eating in the wrong sequence, and eating at the wrong time. The first two points, at least, are valid. Maimonides further noted that even good foods will be poorly digested if the stomach becomes engorged with them. Physicians preached throughout the Middle Ages that "a large supper imposes the greatest punishment on the stomach."

The medical dangers of overeating are illustrated in modern times by the case of a forty-four-year-old Reno physician whose lower esophagus and stomach split on Thanksgiving Day when he vomited violently from having eaten too much turkey dinner. He died of the medical complications of this tragedy by New Year's Day.

Many car owners know that if you overfill your crankcase with oil, you may blow a seal. But most eaters think that the human stomach can be crammed with impunity. Thus, the latest *Guinness Book of World Records,* in a chapter titled "Human Achievements," notes that various men and women throughout the world have downed:

- 2,380 cold baked beans, one at a time, in thirty minutes;
- 424 Little Neck clams in eight minutes;
- Seventeen bananas in two minutes; and
- Thirteen raw eggs (without shells) in 2.2 seconds.

The last record is reminiscent of the scene in the film *Cool Hand Luke* in which Paul Newman consumes fifty hardboiled eggs in sixty minutes, while his fellow prisoners cheer and take bets on whether he can do it.

Other real-life eating records include one set by a Swedish woman, Miss Helge Anderson, who has been drinking forty pints of water daily since 1922 — a condition known as polydipsia or pathological thirst. A similar, rare condition is bulimia or morbid desire to eat. Those who are afflicted have been known to spend fifteen hours a day eating.

A most unusual eating record was set in 1977 by Monsieur "Mangetout" Lotito, who consumed a bicycle in fifteen days in the form of bits of rubber tire and metal filings. *Guinness* will accept no further entries in this category. In the interest of public safety, *Guinness* also refuses to list records of consumption of more than two quarts of beer, and none involving liquor, or such items as live ants, goldfish, marshmallows, or raw eggs in shells.

The average American, who does not set any world records, each year consumes 56 pounds of fats and oils, 126 pounds of beef, 129 pounds of sugar, 5 pounds of additives, 8½ pounds of salt, and the equivalent of 295 twelve-ounce cans of soft drinks. Much of the sugar, one-third of the salt, and most of the additives are hidden in processed foods. Some critics would say it is healthier to consume a bicycle.

Others would call such critics "health nuts." The United States Public Health Service simply recommends that adults reduce consumption of fats, cholesterol, salt, and sugar.

The amount of food you eat affects not only how you digest your food but, according to some theories, how long you live. It has long been known that rats whose diets are restricted live longer than those given unlimited access to food. Other animal studies suggest that dietary restriction instituted in adulthood rejuvenates the immune system, which protects the body against infection and possibly against certain cancers, thereby increasing chances of survival for mice, if not for men.

Other evidence that low caloric intake increases longevity comes from studies of populations like the people of Abkhasia in the Caucasus region of Russia. These people, who appear to live unusually long and healthy lives, for decades have been overrun by scientists wanting to know how they do it. One way is that they remain fit and healthy through vigorous physical exercise. They also avoid tobacco, and eat and drink sparingly. They chew their food slowly and consume relatively little meat or salt, and few eggs — all of which are suspected to cause or worsen blood vessel disease. Moreover, few Abkhasians are obese.

A somewhat contradictory result comes from a study of normal human aging being conducted by the Gerontology Research Center of the National Institute on Aging, in Baltimore, Maryland. There were higher survival rates among subjects in this study who were heavy, though not obese. Dr. Reubin Andres of the National Institute of Aging recently wrote that major population studies fail to show that being ten to thirty percent overweight increases your risk of death.

Other longevity studies dating as far back as 1889 have recommended everything from wearing porous underwear to picking the right grandparents. All have recommended moderation in the use of alcohol and tobacco, and in the amount you eat. People who abuse alcohol and tobacco and overstuff themselves, suffer digestive consequences ranging from simple indigestion to fatal liver disease, as described in later chapters.

The *kind* of food you eat also has profound effects on

your digestive tract. Thomas Jefferson, who ate a lot of vegetables, little meat, and moderate amounts of spirits and strong wine, wrote to a friend in 1819: "I have been blest with organs of digestion which accept and concoct without ever murmuring whatever the palate chooses to consign to them, and I have not yet lost a tooth by age." (S.N. Randolph, *The Domestic Life of Thomas Jefferson*, Charlottesville, Va.: University of Virginia Press, 1978) Jefferson surpassed the eighteenth-century life expectancy of fifty years or less and lived well into his eighties. He also remained mentally and physically active throughout his life.

Certain foods can cause not only digestive problems such as diarrhea, nausea, or a general sick feeling, but reactions like headache, hives, and asthma, and can even send the body into shock. For example, some people have an enzyme deficiency that makes them unable to digest milk and milk products, and other people are allergic to bread, wheat, gluten, fish and seafood, eggs, and chocolate. If sensitivity to these foods causes such problems, you will notice them three to four hours after eating. One way to identify the offending food is to ask your doctor about going on an allergy elimination diet. The late Dr. Herman Tarnower described one way to do this in *The Complete Scarsdale Medical Diet* (N.Y.: Rawson, 1978). For three full days you eat nothing but oatmeal for breakfast; lamb chops, buttered carrots and rice for lunch and supper; and drink only water. If, after three days, you are still having diarrhea and other symptoms, food allergy is probably not the cause. But if the symptoms subside during the three days, start adding foods one at a time that commonly cause allergies until diarrhea or other symptoms recur.

The American Digestive Disease Society has designed six dietary plans that recognize diet as a contributing factor to digestive diseases, and help individuals with digestive problems achieve some control over their diet and their disease. The plans are designed to provide good nutrition during flare-ups of ulcers, gallbladder problems, intestinal gas, inflammatory bowel disease and diverticulitis, irritable bowel syndrome, and inability to digest milk. The plans offer a diet of several basic foods that can be eaten safely even when you are feeling terrible, and show you how to incorporate additional foods into your diet as you begin to feel better (see Appendix A).

Even when healthy, many people cannot tolerate certain foods. One offender is monosodium glutamate (MSG), a flavor enhancer which many chefs use with a heavy hand in Chinese food. The reaction it causes — Chinese restaurant syndrome (CRS) — includes burning sensations in the neck and forearms, chest pain, and headaches. A newer and perhaps more serious form of CRS causes nausea, stomach cramps, dehydration, and diarrhea. This condition will be discussed in Chapter 7.

Other substances that can cause trouble for the digestive tract include spicy foods such as pepper, mustard, garlic, horseradish, paprika, quinine water, vinegary salad dressings, pickled vegetables, and caffeine, a dietary staple for millions of Americans who consume tea, chocolate, soft drinks, and especially, coffee. According to coffee industry people, over half the United States population aged ten and older drinks coffee. These individuals drink an average of 3.2 cups a day, although an estimated five million people drink more than ten cups daily. Over time, coffee and other mild caustics can damage the lining of the stomach severely enough to cause corrosive gastritis (see Chapter 5). Dr. William Lukash, White House physician to Presidents Carter, Ford, and Nixon, has conducted research showing that thirty percent of about two hundred coffee drinkers in the study had digestive diseases directly caused by this habit. Coffee use has recently been linked — statistically at least — to cancer of the pancreas (see Chapter 11), although there is considerable controversy over this finding.

Actor John Barrymore once said, "America is the country where you buy a lifetime supply of aspirin for one dollar and use it up in two weeks." The amount of aspirin consumed in the United States totals more than twenty-seven million pounds a year. Aspirin — which typically consists of five grains (or about three hundred milligrams) of acetylsalicylic acid combined with ordinary starch and pressed into tablet form — can cause gastritis (inflammation of the stomach lining). If aspirin use is heavy, it can also cause gastrointestinal bleeding and aggravate ulcers. When aspirin is taken with or soon after drinking alcohol — to relieve a hangover headache, for example — the irritation it causes to the stomach lining is even worse because both substances are caustic. Drinking a cup of coffee on the morning of a hangover adds a third offender.

The American Digestive Disease Society says that alcohol causes more digestive problems than any other item in the average diet, including the most serious forms of damage to the liver, pancreas, and stomach. In 1975, Americans drank an average of 1.98 gallons of whiskey, 1.70 gallons of wine, and 21.6 gallons of beer for every man, woman, and child. By another accounting, two-thirds of the adult population consumes at least three alcoholic beverages per week, and half of these people drink considerably more. If you add the amount of alcohol consumed by an estimated ten million problem drinkers in the United States, you come up with a lot of liquor and a lot of damage — all forms of which this book will discuss.

"Junk food disease" is the latest gastrointestinal offender to arrive on the American scene. This has been described as a form of marginal malnutrition that causes severe abdominal pains, mainly among adolescents. It resembles beriberi, a severe vitamin B_1 deficiency found in the Orient among people who eat only rice. The diet of a junk-food-disease victim typically consists of soft drinks, pastries, candy, potato chips, and pretzels, supplemented, perhaps, by some milk, french fries, and hamburgers. In medical circles, there is a controversy about whether junk food disease, in fact, exists. But since there are few studies of adolescent nutrition, this controversy will not be resolved soon.

If automobiles brought fast food to us, and us to fast food, the postindustrial era now has a new problem: what to do when you pull into your motel at 3:00 A.M. and all the fast-food places are closed? *Penthouse* magazine provided the answer in its February 1981 issue: it published recipes for motel-emergency delicacies like stick-to-your-ribs rarebit and fish à la manifold. The rarebit recipe goes like this:

Crumble two bags of Cheetos into a shoe. Add enough warm water to form the Cheetos crumbs into a thick paste. Place the paste-filled shoe on a warmed-up TV until the insides bubble. Use the leftover Cheetos to scoop the paste out of the shoe, like fondue.

Fish à la manifold is a bit more intricate. You take frozen fish sticks and wrap them securely in aluminum foil, then wire the package to your car's exhaust manifold. Drive five miles at most, lift the hood, and smell the aroma of baking fish. When a man in Orlando, Florida heard about the fish recipe, he said, "Hey, I'm going to try that!"

Good nutrition has never been adequately defined and, as the American Digestive Disease Society points out, ". . . there is a balanced diet for *each* of us, but not for all of us at the same time."

Nevertheless, there is a set of dietary goals, recommended in 1977 by the Senate Select Committee on Nutrition and Human Needs (known as the McGovern Committee) and later adopted by the Departments of Agriculture, and Health and Human Services. These goals are designed to reduce mortality from heart disease, colon and breast cancer, high blood pressure, obesity, diabetes, arteriosclerosis, and cirrhosis of the liver. The Committee advises that Americans who do not need special diets limit their intake of foods that are linked to killer diseases, and:

- Eat a variety of foods.
- Eat fewer calories.
- Eat less fat, saturated fat, and cholesterol.
- Eat more foods with adequate starch and fiber.
- Eat less refined and processed sugar.
- Eat less salt.
- Drink less alcohol.

The kinds of foods you eat are important, but so is the way you eat them. A pleasant dining atmosphere with candlelight and congenial company can help you digest your food, whereas family fights at mealtime wage on in your gut. Contact between family members is often inescapable at meals. If you are forced to take food with someone with whom you are in conflict, mealtime may become an orgy of indigestion, stomach cramps, diarrhea, nausea, and vomiting. "It's enough to make you sick," the saying goes, and indeed, it may be.

To escape family mealtime madness, make up, eat out, or move out. But realize that eating out exposes you to new hazards, namely the "eating out syndrome," caused by eating strange food in a strange setting at a strange hour. All this may upset your digestion. You may eat more than you are accustomed to, at a different pace than you are accustomed to, with more drinks and wine than you are accustomed to. If eating out leaves you with late-night gas pain, heartburn, and a feeling of queasiness, consider making some changes the next time you go to a restaurant: a little less bread between courses, a little more restraint on the amount you eat, and a little more thought to how the foods you order will agree with you. The object is to keep restaurant eating patterns more in line with daily eating habits.

Whatever and whenever you eat, try to pay attention to your food. Too many people eat like fugitives — alone and on the run — perhaps not even sitting down, perhaps not looking away from the newspaper propped up in front of them. Weight Watchers, a support group that helps fat people lose weight, advises their members not to interrupt their eating by television, reading, or even by conversation. In his *Scarsdale Medical Diet* book, Dr. Herman Tarnower advocates the Tarnower Eating Philosophy: ". . . the simplest dish should be viewed and treated with admiration and respect. A scrambled egg or a hamburger can be beautiful. . . . The true enjoyment is gone once the food leaves the mouth. Chew, chew, chew."

An earlier version of the Tarnower Eating Philosophy was advocated by Horace Fletcher, a late-nineteenth-century businessman from Ohio. Fletcher believed that his countrymen ate too much, and so suggested that they chew each mouthful fifty or sixty times. This was an embellishment of an earlier recommendation by Lord William Gladstone, a nineteenth-century British statesman who thought that the reason humans have thirty-two teeth is that nature intended us to chew each mouthful of food thirty-two times (once for each tooth). Fletcher later raised it to two hundred to three hundred times, and even suggested chewing whiskey. Fletcherizing had several advantages. It made it unnecessary to swallow food — it just ran down your gullet. Fletcherizing was also a way to cut calories: because it took so long, there was no time to overeat. Fletcher later advised that the eater chew face down, so that "the tongue hangs perpendicular in the mouth."

In an article published in *Cosmopolitan* magazine in 1908, Elbert Hubbard, an apostle of Fletcher, wrote that fletcherizing a martini makes it taste, after two or three small sips, just like kerosene. Psychologist William James tried fletcherizing for three months and said, "It nearly killed me."

Even West Point took to fletcherizing. Thirty officers-to-be were assigned to the study. When the project was explained to them, six deserted. But those who remained became more vigorous and thinner as the weeks passed. At the end of the experiment, the War Department reported that "they developed a marked readiness to kill."

Meanwhile, Fletcher himself did poorly. He took nothing but liquids, and eventually became constipated. But this did not bother Fletcher. He considered his condition part of a "natural sterilizing process" and sent a sample stool — when one finally emerged — to a federal laboratory as a gift.

Horace Fletcher's health code might not have survived had it not been for Upton Sinclair, who immortalized fletcherizing in these simple lines:

> Nature will castigate
> Those who don't masticate.

The ancient Greeks and Romans knew another way to eat pleasurably. They reclined on their left sides while dining, probably because this position encouraged stomach acids to flow and aid digestion. The eating habits of the people of Abkhasia, mentioned earlier, are even better. One study shows that good nutrition is evident in people who like a variety of foods, who enjoy sharing it with others, who are mentally and physically active, self-disciplined and secure, and well integrated into their communities. In contrast, depression, loneliness, immaturity, and anxiety have an overall negative effect on nutrition. Thus, while choosing and digesting the right food is important, the spirit in which you eat may be even more crucial. In other words, good nutrition — and good digestion — may be a way of living a positive, enjoyable life. Hippocrates, who lived at a time when foods were used to soothe stomachs, wrote, "Thy food shall be thy remedy." And thy downfall.

PART II

Common Complaints

CHAPTER 5

My Stomach Hurts

Indigestion

IN HIS BOOK *Mortal Lessons: Notes on the Art of Surgery* (N.Y.: Simon & Schuster, 1974), Richard Selzer, author and physician, tells of the aweto — a caterpillarlike inhabitant of New Zealand which refuses all nourishment except the seed of a certain fungus. But the seed, once eaten, germinates and grows so quickly that the aweto cannot expel it — either way. In Selzer's words:

> Soon the malevolent fungus can be seen emerging from the mouth of the aweto, elongating, dividing, thrusting spurs through the aweto's brain. Now the aweto has the look of an anguished elk. It is thus, crammed and bursting, that the aweto dies, its corpse a mere fingerling upon the burgeoning meal-beast.

The meal-monsters you consume do not consume you in turn. Nor, on the other hand, do they pass unnoticed.

Most of the time, when your stomach hurts, it is due to indigestion, otherwise known as dyspepsia, upset stomach, "acid" indigestion, or plain indigestion. But it means only one thing: you are not digesting your food properly. By contrast, hunger pangs are simply the muscular contractions of an empty stomach.

Indigestion ranges from mild discomfort in the midriff

area *after* a meal, to a bloated feeling, to the burning sensation of "acid" indigestion, to more severe abdominal pain. Indigestion may also cause nausea and vomiting, belching, constipation, or diarrhea. When you get indigestion, you have most likely overtaxed your digestive system by eating too much, eating too fast, or eating foods that are too fatty, spicy, or rich. Still, nobody knows the exact cause of this postprandial distress. It may be caused by irritation from stomach secretions, or by the discomfort of a stomach stretched from a large meal. Sometimes indigestion is a sign of something more serious. Call a doctor immediately if indigestion is severe and is accompanied by:

- ◆ Difficulty in breathing.
- ◆ Sudden nausea or vomiting.
- ◆ Fainting.
- ◆ Rapid heartbeats.
- ◆ Heavy sweating.
- ◆ A cold, clammy feeling.

Sometimes heart attacks are at first mistaken for indigestion. But indigestion is common and heart attacks are not, especially under the age of forty.

When indigestion occurs frequently, especially after an upsetting experience or during a period of stress, it may have emotional roots as well. Indigestion often strikes during the stresses of exam week, job hunts, premarital jitters, and deadlines. A few years ago, it also struck some people who saw the film *The Exorcist*. They flocked to their doctors afterward with stomach upsets that they thought were caused by evil forces or demons in their bowels. Aside from these occasional ills, studies show that people who have frequent bouts of indigestion tend to be nervous, depressed, and anxious.

Anxiety — a vague uneasiness with no apparent cause — can stimulate the stomach to secrete more acid than is needed for normal digestion. Nervous, depressed people may belch a lot because their nervousness causes them to swallow air, and this increases the feeling of uncomfortable inner pressure in their stomachs. They tend to eat odd foods at odd hours, get little sleep, and have lifestyles as erratic as their eating habits.

If indigestion results from the way you eat and live, so does its cure. Persistent indigestion, or indigestion accompanied by severe abdominal pain, should be checked by a physician to make sure that a more serious disorder is not involved. But most cases of indigestion — even the kinds that persist for years — you can treat yourself. Specifically:

◆ Give your stomach a rest. The problem will probably "cure" itself if you stop eating for several hours, and then resume with bland foods.

◆ Avoid coffee, tea, smoking, and alcohol. They irritate the stomach, and alcohol causes it to produce more acid.

◆ If possible, avoid aspirin and aspirin-containing medications: aspirin damages the stomach lining.

◆ If you must take aspirin, take it with a glass of water to keep it from sticking to a "dry" stomach, or take it with an antacid or with food.

◆ Try natural remedies. Lie on your side or stretch out flat, stomach down. Or you might feel better standing or walking. Experiment to see which remedy works best for you.

◆ Loosen tight-fitting clothing. For example, remove panty hose and tight jeans, and undo your belt.

◆ Contrary to popular opinion, milk is not an effective antacid. It relieves "acid" indigestion for only about fifteen minutes — then it stimulates the stomach to produce even more acid.

A bewildering array of antacids — over five hundred different types — are on the market. These products help some people if taken thirty minutes to an hour after a meal. One antacid, sodium bicarbonate (baking soda), should be used only occasionally. Its commercial forms include Alka-Seltzer and Bromo-Seltzer. Although sodium bicarbonate neutralizes stomach acid, many physicians advise against prolonged use because it may be absorbed into the bloodstream through the walls of the stomach, making the blood more alkaline. This, in turn, may stimulate the stomach to produce even more acid in a kind of "rebound" reaction. In addition, sodium bicarbonate has a high salt content that may be harmful to people with heart disease and / or high blood pressure. An antacid with a low salt content such as Riopan should be taken instead. Finally, antacids that fizz do no good for an already irritated stomach lining.

There are, however, antacids that neutralize stomach juices without unbalancing body chemistry. These are the nonabsorbable antacids: Maalox, Gelusil, and Mylanta, to name a few. The liquid form of these antacids works better because it coats the esophagus and stomach. Antacid tablets are handy to carry around for emergencies, but will do little good unless you chew them thoroughly. Swallowed whole, they can cause intestinal obstruction.

Nonabsorbable antacids usually contain aluminum or magnesium. The former tends to cause constipation, and the latter, diarrhea, so experiment to see which one works best for you. Or try switching from one type to another to offset these side effects. Antacids containing magnesium may be harmful to people with kidney disease, and should be taken only under a doctor's supervision. Other antacids that contain calcium carbonate (better known as chalk) may produce a slight "rebound" effect if used continually, that is, more than four times a day. In addition, antacids containing calcium carbonate tend to cause constipation.

When indigestion is caused by emotional stress, antacids can prevent acid damage to the stomach, but cannot provide an ultimate solution to the problem. If "upset stomachs" seem to precede exams, job hunts, social events, income tax deadlines, or dental appointments, you need to recognize the source of stress (and indigestion) and overcome it. If your symptoms then improve, you will know the next time similar circumstances arise how best to take care of your stomach. There is nothing wrong with antacids, *per se,* as long as they are not a way to avoid finding and facing the real cause of your stomach upsets.

Indigestion is easier to prevent than to cure:

◆ Find out what upsets your stomach and avoid it. Do you get indigestion after eating fried foods, milk, certain kinds of meat, spicy foods, or fruit? Or do you get indigestion after an emotionally upsetting experience?

♦ Do you get indigestion after stuffing yourself with food? Try this exercise: push your chair away from the table before your plate is empty, or eat smaller portions in the first place.

♦ Do you have erratic habits, keep irregular hours, get too little sleep, eat at odd times, or eat bizarre foods? Try to change these facets of your lifestyle.

Do you get stomach upsets after long and jarring car rides? Such troubles may be caused by the tensions of driving, which have been reported to inhibit gastric movement and secretion. The meal sits in the stomach, creating a sense of nausea and heaviness. You should start a long car trip with a light meal, or wait one or two hours after a heavy one. During the trip, avoid fatty, rich foods.

Indigestion-on-wheels is another example of the stresses that modern civilization places on your unsuspecting stomach and bowels. You can replace a car that has suffered too much wear and tear. But when your body's engine goes bad, you cannot trade it in for a new model.

Heartburn

Also known as pyrosis, inner fire, or gastroesophageal reflux, heartburn is a symptom, not a disease. It is characterized by a steady, burning pain at the tip of your breastbone that occurs when your stomach is full. It strikes thirty minutes to two hours after a meal, and is made worse by lying down. Heartburn pain may travel into your arms, and make you think you are having a heart attack even though the problem has nothing to do with your heart.

Heartburn occurs when the muscular ring at the junction of your esophagus and stomach — the esophageal valve — fails to close properly and stomach juices back up into the esophagus. Unlike the stomach, the esophagus has no natural protection. When stomach secretions backflow, a hot sensation occurs in the pit of your stomach or just beneath your breastbone.

Sometimes, stomach acids cause esophagitis, an inflammation of the esophagus. It may also become inflamed if you have hiatus hernia — a protrusion of part of the stomach into your chest cavity. Hiatus hernia was once considered the major cause of chronic heartburn, but no longer. Many adults with hiatus hernia do not have heartburn (see Chapter 9). These same digestive juices may also irritate and inflame the lining of your stomach and cause gastritis. Or these acids may cause ulcers — craterlike sores in your stomach or the first part of your small intestine (see Chapter 9).

Conversely, people who have gastritis or ulcers tend to develop heartburn. Pregnant women frequently suffer from heartburn, in part because of the pressures that the growing fetus exerts on the esophageal sphincter. The afflicted also include people with certain "heartburn habits" like belching, chewing gum, swallowing air, sucking on hard candies, smoking, eating too fast, eating too much, bending over or slumping when the stomach is full, and taking naps after meals. Overeating distends the stomach, and naps give gravity a hand in allowing gastric juices to flow back into the esophagus. And alcohol, aspirin, coffee, tea, cola drinks, fruit juices, chocolate, and greasy or heavily spiced foods provoke heartburn because they cause increased motor activity and acid secretion, or otherwise irritate the stomach.

In one study, the majority of forty-six patients with heartburn had poor eating habits. They downed great quantities of liquids with meals, drank carbonated beverages, and in various other ways overdistended their stomachs. They ate their meals under tension, rushed through meals, argued, and gulped down food so that they could get the next word in. These same patients tended to be extremely tense, resentful, argumentative individuals who said they got "burnt up" easily and had trouble "swallowing" certain situations.

About half of all people who complain of heartburn are air swallowers. They are nervous individuals who breathe too quickly, gasp, and sigh, rather than inhale at an easy, regular pace. During periods of anxiety, they have been known to swallow up to several liters of air in a short span of time. Air swallowers may develop a "stomach bubble" of air that has been swallowed but not belched or passed through the bowel as intestinal gas. The trapped air causes the stomach to bloat and distend, and creates pressure that weakens the esophageal valve. This gas bubble may force gastric juices upward, and cause heartburn. Cigarette smoking also contributes to heartburn, as does coffee, stress, and eating out of habit rather than necessity. A recent study shows that people who swallow cold drinks, ice cream, and other cold foods too quickly sometimes develop sharp pains in the chest. The pain has nothing to do with the heart, and apparently is caused by dilation of the esophagus to twice its normal size by the sudden introduction of cold food and drink.

How to handle heartburn:

♦ Don't recline after eating. Sit up or stand, and let gravity send acids back into the stomach.

♦ Sleep with your head raised at least four inches.

♦ Don't eat or drink for two hours before bedtime.

♦ Avoid the common irritants like alcohol, aspirin, coffee, and tea.

♦ Eat smaller portions of food, increasing the number of meals if you are not overweight. If you are overweight, slim down.

♦ Consider the possibility that the way you react to emotional stress might predispose you to heartburn, especially if you tend to swallow air.

♦ Remember that, contrary to myth, milk does not help heartburn. It has the opposite effect because it increases gastric secretions.

Antacids are the primary treatment for heartburn. Take them about an hour after meals and at bedtime, or more often if heartburn symptoms persist. Many doctors recommend the nonabsorbable antacids like Maalox, Gelusil, Mylanta, or Riopan. Antacids that have a high sodium content, like sodium bicarbonate (Alka-Seltzer), may give quick relief, but shouldn't be used repeatedly for heartburn even if you are otherwise healthy. And high-sodium antacids should be used only on a physician's advice if you have heart diseases, high blood pressure, or are pregnant. Liquid antacids work better than tablets because they coat greater areas of the esophagus and stomach. Tablets must be fletcherized (chewed well) to be effective. Keep the antacid solution chilled. It tastes better that way. Clinical trials of a new drug, cimetidine, which is used to treat ulcers, are underway to determine if it also relieves heartburn, but the Food and Drug Administration has not, as of this writing, approved the marketing of cimetidine for that use.

Pain caused by heart disease is generally sharper than that caused by heartburn, and may occur after exercising. Heartburn pain, on the other hand, often follows a heavy meal and is worsened by lying down or bending over. If, in addition to heartburn, you have trouble swallowing food, or vomit black or bloody material, or pass bloody or tarlike black stools, or feel "heartburn" pain clear through to your back, you may have a serious problem that needs a physician's immediate attention. But most of the time, you can control heartburn, like so many other stomach ailments, on your own.

Motion Sickness

The term *motion sickness* was first used in 1881 to describe what sometimes happens to people when they travel by car, coach, train, swing, and sea, not to mention elephant and camel. The most familiar form of this problem is seasickness, or *mal de mer*. Some famous people have reportedly suffered from seasickness, including Noah, Julius Caesar, St. Paul, and Charles Darwin. Lord Nelson's doctors were not able to cure his seasickness, although it never lasted very long. And Lawrence of Arabia got sick whenever he climbed atop a camel, appropriately referred to as the "ship of the desert."

In modern times, astronauts have succumbed. During the fourth Skylab mission, in November 1973, astronauts Gerald Carr, Edward Gibson, and William Pogue tried to conceal the fact that Pogue had vomited during a brief spell of motion sickness about eight hours after launching. The following conversation then took place aboard Skylab:

CARR: Well, Bill, I think we better tell the truth tonight since we're going to have a fecal vomitus bag to turn in, although I guess we could throw that down the trash airlock and forget the whole thing. . . . Let's do that then. We won't mention the barf.

GIBSON: . . . You know damn well that every manager in NASA would probably, under his breath, want you to do that.

The astronauts did not realize that an onboard recorder was taping their conversation! Mission Control informed the three astronauts that they had made "a fairly serious error in judgment." According to a report in *Medical World News,* Carr agreed that it was "a dumb decision." Actually, the astronauts had redeemed themselves before Mission Control chided them by deciding not to dump the vomitus bag.

Not even animals are immune to "motion sickness": horses, cows, monkeys, seals, sheep, cats, dogs, and even fish have been reported to get seasick. The owner of one fish hatchery loaded some cod in a tank aboard a boat to transport them to another location. The fish had been fed about an hour earlier. As soon as the boat put to sea, all the feed they had eaten ended up on the bottom of the tank. Today it is common practice to make fish fast before transporting them.

The classic symptoms of motion sickness include queasy stomach, heavy salivation, pallor, cold sweating, nausea, and vomiting. Motion sickness also causes indifference to social surroundings, depression, a wish to be left alone and / or to die, and, in the case of the Skylab IV astronauts, acute embarrassment.

Much of what is known about motion sickness in humans was learned during World War II when sea- and airsickness were matters of tactics and strategy. One colonel took his men out to sea off Virginia Beach in amphibious landing craft to prove they could fight upon landing. They sailed six miles and were violently seasick. As the craft returned to shore, a line of skeptical generals and admirals awaited the results. The colonel told his men that if they did not charge through that line of brass, they would take another boat trip! The final report showed that troops could probably cross the English Channel and remain fit to fight.

At this time, there was much concern about seasickness and how it might affect combat effectiveness in the Normandy Invasion. War correspondent Ernie Pyle tells in his book *Brave Men* (N.Y.: Holt and Co., 1943) what happened:

> The night before sailing we were instructed to take two anti-seasickness capsules before breakfast the next day, and follow them up with one every four hours throughout the voyage. . . . Well, we took the first two and they almost killed us. The capsules had a strong sleeping powder in them, and by noon all the Army personnel aboard were in a drugged stupor. Fortunately the Navy, being proud, didn't take any, so somebody was left to run the ship. The capsules not only put us to sleep but they constricted our throats, made our mouths bone-dry and dilated the pupils of our eyes until we could hardly see. When we recovered from this insidious jag, along toward evening, we threw our seasickness medicine away, and after that we felt fine.

The "insidious jag" was caused by a drug called, in military parlance, Motion Sickness Preventive — United States Army Development Type. It contained one grain of sodium amytal, $1/300$ grain of scopolamine hydrobromide, and $1/400$ grain of atropine sulfate, enough to put anybody to sleep. After the invasion, the chief surgeon for the European Theater of Operations received a report stating that the drug apparently had not reduced the incidence of seasickness. A true test, he added, had not been possible because of "operational conditions" and the "delegating (of) medical functions, such as the administration of potent drugs, to untrained lay personnel in the Army."

Various studies show that in more ordinary circumstances, the rate of motion sickness for humans is about:

- Sixty percent on life rafts in the ocean.
- Twenty-five to thirty percent during the first days of an Atlantic crossing.
- Three to four percent in trains and cars.
- One-half percent on an airliner.

But when motion sickness strikes on any one airplane, the incidence rises to eight percent because of the power of suggestion. In recent years, however, jet airliners have been flying at higher, smoother altitudes, and motion sickness has become less of a problem.

Individuals vary in their susceptibility. Although it is known that repeated or continued exposure to motion helps most people adapt, some never get their "car legs" or "sea legs." A five-year-old girl got carsick in the back seat but not in the front. State of mind also plays an important role. One teenaged girl had such fear of flying that she threw up on the ramp entering the plane. Fifteen years earlier, the girl's mother had thrown up in the terminal as soon as she caught sight of the plane! Some yachtsmen do fine in small boats, but turn green when they sail on an oceanliner. Seasickness also depends upon the type and construction of the vessel, and on its speed and course relative to prevailing swell conditions.

The physical mechanism of motion sickness is not well understood, although it appears to have something to do with tilting of the fluid in your inner ear. The balance-control system in your brain — which tells you whether you're standing up straight, turning, or bending over — turns itself off because it has too much sensory input from violent movement and visual disturbance. Motion sickness is more likely to affect people when they sit up than when they lie down. According to another theory, motion sickness occurs when the information your ears and other senses receive does not conform to what your senses *expect* to receive, based on previous experience.

These findings suggest some ways to control motion sickness:

◆ Rest up before a trip. Fatigue worsens motion sickness.

◆ Try the repetition remedy. Take frequent short trips in a car, for example, to accustom your balance system to driving.

◆ Jog or swim. People who engage in these sports are less prone to motion sickness because their balance systems are accustomed to movement.

◆ In a car or train, focus on distant scenery rather than

on the dashboard or nearby telephone poles whizzing by.

◆ At sea, remain on deck, gaze at the distant horizon, and keep busy. Chipping paint from a bulkhead is considered the best cure for seasickness in young sailors.

◆ If you're in the tail of a plane, switch to a seat over the wheels, because the tail portion moves more than the body of the plane.

◆ Wherever you are, hold your head still. Brace it against the back of your seat, and if you move it, do so slowly.

◆ Avoid reading, tobacco smoke, and unpleasant odors — they can make motion sickness worse.

◆ Since diet plays an important role in motion sickness, don't eat or drink for an hour before the trip, and don't snack in the car.

◆ Remember, one drink might help since alcohol is a tranquilizer, but more will stimulate your balance mechanism and produce a sense of motion, making the problem worse.

◆ Ask your doctor to recommend a drug for motion sickness, or try an over-the-counter product (Dramamine and Bonine are frequently used). Bear in mind that these medications may cause drowsiness, and should be taken twenty to sixty minutes before departure.

Dozens of drugs help control motion sickness by acting on the central nervous system. They can raise your resistance to motion sickness, but will not work in extreme situations. Nor will they help when taken orally after vomiting has started. At that point, a doctor must administer them by injection. Antiemetic suppositories, which stop you from vomiting after about thirty minutes, are also available. Another new delivery system consists of a seasickness drug, scopolamine, that is stuck behind the ear. The drug is contained in a device called "the patch," which is about the size of a dime and a few millimeters thick. The medication is absorbed directly through the skin behind the ear.

But no delivery system on earth could induce astronauts on the second Skylab mission to take motion-sickness drugs. They refused until severe symptoms, including vomiting, had occurred. The reason for this refusal, Dr. Charles A. Berry told *Medical World News*, is that astronauts have a certain machismo that "prevents them from wanting to use any kind of crutch such as a pill."

Later, Dr. Berry and other NASA flight surgeons tried to convince the astronauts to take a motion-sickness tablet, wait an hour, and then move their heads back and forth forty times a minute for up to half an hour. Ground tests had shown that these exercises help men adapt to motion in a revolving room for twenty-four hours. But the astronauts, who remained skeptical of the relationship between queasy stomachs and head movements, took four days to adapt, and several more days to replace body fluids and salts lost through vomiting.

Nausea and Vomiting

Nausea is the unpleasant urge to throw up. In a sense, vomiting is a "cure" for nausea. Throughout the ages, people have deliberately induced vomiting to rid themselves of poisons or too much food in the stomach. The Romans made vomiting a social grace so they could enjoy food at night-long revels. They did it by pressing a finger against the soft palate or by tickling that area with a scented feather. Later *lori vomitorium*, or greased probes, were inserted as far down as the esophagus to induce vomiting.

Some other ways to make yourself vomit include drinking syrup of ipecac or eating activated charcoal. The annals of college fraternity history include accounts of freshmen forced to swallow an oyster with a string tied around it to induce vomiting. Once the downward slither of the oyster is interrupted and the creature is pulled back up the esophagus, you are sure to vomit, but the finger-down-the-throat method is far safer.

There are times when you should *not* induce vomiting — when someone has swallowed a strong acid or alkali or other corrosive substance. There are also times when you simply *cannot* induce vomiting. You go through all the motions of vomiting — the lower part of your stomach contracts violently, and the pyloric, or "exit" valve to the duodenum remains firmly shut — but nothing comes up. These "dry heaves" usually occur after about ten minutes of vomiting, when there is nothing *left* in the stomach to bring up. At that point, you may vomit some brownish yellow bile from the duodenum. This is no cause for alarm. It usually just means that the duodenum is contracting with the stomach.

The causes of involuntary nausea and vomiting include eating too much, drinking too much, and eating contaminated food or poison. You may also vomit if you react badly to certain drugs such as antibiotics, digitalis, or aspirin, or if you are allergic to certain foods. Other conditions that may cause nausea include pregnancy, stomach flu, kidney disease, heart disease, concussion, diabetes, certain infections, migraine headaches, hyperthyroidism, and a wide variety of digestive diseases.

Psychogenic vomiting, or throwing up for emotional reasons, may occur if you experience sudden shock, fright, or bad news, or if you are under severe emotional stress. Consider the case of an eight-year-old girl whose chronic vomiting resulted from a tragic accident. One day after going to the store for soft drinks and cupcakes, she and her mother were struck by a car as they crossed the street. Gail suffered minor physical injuries, but her mother died en route to the hospital. For the next few months, Gail threw up her breakfast every morning. A doctor examined her and could find no physical cause for her vomiting. The doctor then learned that during the accident, Gail's mother had been thrown into the air and had landed on Gail's stomach. Because she believed her hunger had caused her mother's death, she threw up every time she got hungry. Only when her doctor helped her understand the emotional causes of her vomiting was she able to stop.

Vomiting serves an emotional purpose when it provokes someone's concern or anger, a phenomenon known as "secondary gain." A child may vomit in response to a situation he fears, such as the first day of school. If the vomiting continues, it can become a way of avoiding the second, third, and fourth days of school. One thirteen-year-old girl began vomiting regularly — and was even hospitalized several times — when she discovered that her illness kept her mother from leaving home and divorcing her father. Battered children tend to vomit for days after being beaten. Conversely, many children learn that if they vomit or have abdominal cramps, they will be held in a warm embrace.

Many of the patients in one study of psychogenic vomiters lived with people toward whom they felt enraged. But none of them took steps to remove themselves from these hostile relationships. Most of them seemed unwilling to "cut their losses" by moving away because they had experienced the painful loss of a parent when they were young, and were unwilling to accept a further loss. Significantly, many of the vomiters shared the same house and ate at the same table with the sources of their antagonism. Most of the patients vomited chiefly at mealtime. One woman loathed her husband but felt there was nowhere she could go. She started vomiting within a few weeks of their marriage. Another woman felt guilty because she could not look after her chronically ill mother. She vomited during one visit to her mother and, thereafter, vomited regularly during visits.

Vomiting may also be triggered by the more ordinary stresses of marital discord, mealtime madness, failure to find a job, sexual problems, adjustment to marriage or a new location, the loss of a loved one, or terminal illness in the family.

Another cause of vomiting is morning sickness, the common term for the nausea and vomiting that afflict half of all women who become pregnant. Usually, morning sickness is completely gone by noon, and lasts only through the sixth to twelfth week of pregnancy. But if it continues all day long for days at a time, it may become life-threatening because of food and fluid loss. A physician should treat these cases of *hyperemesis gravidarium,* or excessive vomiting from pregnancy.

Fatigue, distress, and unhappiness can precipitate morning sickness or make it worse. Other explanations for its occurrence include hormone changes or carbohydrate deficiency.

Morning sickness is a uniquely human disorder. Animals do not appear to develop it, even when scientists try to induce it in pregnant laboratory animals. It has been suggested that this may be so because dogs, cats, and other animals do not worry about "another mouth to feed," about losing their figures, or that pregnancy is a punishment for having enjoyed intercourse.

To prevent vomiting:

♦ Eat smaller portions of food.
♦ Avoid drinking large amounts of fluids, especially at mealtimes, and take small sips.
♦ Loosen clothing and get some fresh air.
♦ Relax. Fatigue makes nausea and vomiting worse.
♦ If vomiting persists, see your doctor.
♦ To recuperate from vomiting, put nothing in your stomach for two to three hours after the last bout of nausea and vomiting.
♦ Then try clear, cool beverages such as water, iced tea, or flat gingerale. If you tolerate these well, start solid foods two or three hours later.
♦ Work up slowly to a normal diet, starting with soups, bouillon, Jell-O, applesauce, toast, crackers, and salty foods, and avoid sweets.
♦ Suck on ice chips if nothing else will stay down.
♦ According to one nine-year-old, eat a piece of white-bread toast with no butter, drink a coke with one ice cube, lie on a mattress with no covers, and watch Bugs Bunny reruns!

Dehydration is one of the dangers of vomiting, but it usually takes a day or two to develop, and is more likely to happen if you have diarrhea as well. Infants and children become dehydrated more quickly than adults. Dehydration is a threat if a child under two loses all fluid intake for six hours, if a child between two and ten years old loses all fluid intake for eight to ten hours, or if an adult loses all fluid intake for twelve hours. You should also see a doctor immediately if the vomit appears black or bloody, for it could be a sign of internal bleeding. Aspiration, or inhaling vomit into the windpipe or lungs, is another danger, especially for the unconscious person. To prevent it, keep that person lying stomach down, head turned to the side.

Some people have the ability to ruminate, i.e., to regurgitate undigested food and fluid fifteen to thirty minutes after a meal. Ruminators eat large amounts of food quickly. Then, without conscious intent, they bring their food back up without feeling nauseated, rechew and reswallow it, and profess to enjoy it even more the second time around! Some ruminators regurgitate food fifteen to twenty times within an hour, and stop only when it begins to taste sour.

One man made a career of his ability to ruminate. He appeared at county fairs and swallowed large amounts of water containing live goldfish and a frog, and brought them up on request from the audience. If the spectators asked for the goldfish and the frog happened to come up first, he quickly reswallowed the frog and brought up the goldfish instead.

Rumination is the human equivalent of "chewing cud" in grass-eating animals. The stomachs of ruminant animals have four anatomic chambers. The first two serve as receptacles for food that the animal rechews when it has time to do so.

Rumination commonly occurs in people who have upper gastrointestinal abnormalities, including hiatus hernia, duodenal ulcer, stomach cancer, and weakness of the esophageal valve. In nauseless vomiting, closely related to rumination, certain individuals can bring up the entire contents of their stomachs at will, without effort or discomfort.

The condition achalasia is caused by a severe spasm of the lower esophageal valve, which may result in involuntary regurgitation of food when the esophagus is fully distended. Your chest may feel tight because food is stuck in the esophagus just above the valve. If those muscles do not relax and allow the entrance valve of the stomach to open, food that cannot pass into your stomach may come back up, especially if you are in a horizontal or a head-down position. This condition is relatively rare, and occurs mainly in persons between the ages of thirty and fifty. Often achalasia strikes after severe emotional shock, reflecting a refusal to accept sorrow.

Hangover Gut and Gastritis

Hangover gut or "morning-after" syndrome is the flat tire of the digestive tract. It is the consequence of drinking too much alcohol, which causes more serious digestive problems than any other item in the American diet.

Alcohol is a common cause of acute, or short-term gastritis. The term *gastritis* covers a multitude of stomach ailments, but, strictly speaking, means inflammation of the lining of your stomach. It is usually named after the substance that caused it, for example, alcohol gastritis. According to one theory, alcohol harms the stomach's natural protective barrier — a lining that prevents it from digesting itself. Alcohol also upsets the way your body holds water. And what it does to the rest of your digestive tract will become apparent as you read this book.

For most people, the solution is not to stop drinking, but to learn how to drink intelligently. Here are some suggestions:

♦ Relax or nap before a party. Fatigue increases the rate at which you absorb alcohol. Fear, anger, and sadness have the same effect.
♦ Eat dinner before a party. Food slows the alcohol absorption rate.
♦ Allow time between drinks. A 150-pound person can stay sober by not exceeding one drink (containing an ounce of eighty-proof alcohol), or the equivalent, per hour.
♦ Remember that an ounce of eighty-proof liquor is about equal to a can of beer or 3½ ounces of table wine.
♦ Use water rather than soda as a mixer.
♦ If you are taking any medication, know how it interacts with alcohol. For example, some cough and cold remedies can heighten the effects of alcohol.

The only real remedy for an occasional hangover is rest and the passage of time (about twelve hours will usually do it). Hospital interns and residents, whose job pressures have been known to send them on an occasional binge, stretch out on an examining table the morning after, while a colleague administers a liter of intravenous saline solution! After about forty-five minutes of such reinforcement, they are ready to see patients and perform surgery. The at-home version of this remedy is as follows:

◆ Before retiring, drink water and eat something salty such as soda crackers. Plain water will be less effective in reducing dehydration.

◆ When you wake up, again drink salty fluids such as Gatorade or tomato juice — a quart or more if you aren't too queasy to hold it down. Or eat more soda crackers and sip as much water as you can.

◆ Plan to spend the rest of the morning in bed — your head will hurt less if you do — and let the salt solution rehydrate your body.

◆ Some folks swear that vitamin C, B_{12}, and other nutrients will cure a hangover. However, their bodies are probably craving a restoration of the fluid balance, not specific vitamins.

◆ Taking a "hair-of-the-dog-that-bit-you" remedy (that is, more alcohol) may deaden immediate symptoms, but the relief is only temporary, since morning-after drinking can lead to alcohol dependency.

◆ Avoid mild tranquilizers, sedatives, and antihistamines because they, like alcohol, are depressants that only aggravate a hangover.

◆ Aspirin is a traditional remedy for a hangover. However, like the morning-after cup of coffee, it can irritate your stomach lining. If your head aches so badly that even the cat seems to be stomping, take aspirin with a large glass of water or an antacid to dilute its corrosive effect.

Alcohol and aspirin combined are believed to harm the stomach more than either substance alone. A recent study shows that those brands of aspirin with enteric coatings, which do not dissolve until the drug reaches the intestines, may insulate the stomach from injury. But buffered aspirin tablets offer little or no protection to the stomach.

Other caustics include coffee, spicy foods, strong tea,

quinine water, vinegar salad dressings, and pickled vegetables. Bacterially infected food, food to which you are allergic, poisonous substances, and many drugs, especially steroids and certain antibiotics, can also cause gastritis. Each of these irritants produces different symptoms.

Chronic gastritis is a more serious condition which causes long-term inflammation of the lining of the stomach, often resulting in permanent damage. About fifty percent of all alcoholics suffer from chronic gastritis. The incidence is also high in people with diabetes, high blood pressure, thyroid deficiency, and gastric ulcers. Older people, relatives of diabetics, and people who are very nervous and tense also tend to develop a chronic form of gastritis.

Yet, the real cause of chronic gastritis remains unknown. It is somewhat of a "wastebasket" diagnosis, often cited when no other cause of stomach trouble can be found. Fortunately, the pain of chronic gastritis can be controlled by diet and antacids. The stomach afflicted by gastritis has amazing regenerative capacities, despite our relentless abuse.

"Swimmer's Cramps"

There is an old wives' tale that if you eat before swimming, you will get cramps, double over, and drown. The part about drowning is probably a myth, unless you are a poor swimmer to start with. You are far more likely to lose a race in a swimming competition. When you eat, your heart pumps blood to your stomach and intestines to help you digest food. If you exercise or swim vigorously after eating a large meal, the flow of blood is directed from the stomach and intestines to your muscles. The lack of oxygen-bearing blood can cause the stomach and intestinal muscles to cramp. Exercise after a heavy meal produces other effects as well, including sweating, heart palpitations, and light-headedness. (That is why you sometimes become sleepy or light-headed after a large meal: blood is pumped to your digestive organs and away from other parts of your body, including the brain.)

Several factors determine how long you should wait after meals before exercising. The more you eat, the longer food remains in your stomach. Emotional stress — especially the kind you feel before competition in a sports event — can also slow down the passage of food from your stomach. On the other hand, the more fit you are (and the better your heart can pump blood both to your muscles and to your stomach), the less time you will need to wait before exercising. In general, professional athletes eat a meal three to six hours before an event. The average person who swims for noontime exercise would do better to swim before eating lunch.

Anorexia Nervosa

Though not a digestive disease, per se, this condition is an extremely common and tragic eating disorder that afflicts one in two hundred teenage American girls, and kills from ten to fifteen percent of them. The disorder also strikes teenage boys, although ten to twenty times as many girls are affected.

The typical victim — a twelve- to eighteen-year-old girl - stops eating not because she has lost her appetite, but because she insists that she is too fat. She loses weight, takes on an emaciated, gaunt appearance, and insists that her seventy-pound shrunken body — that long since has stopped menstruating — is "just right." To hasten her weight loss, she may secretly induce vomiting after meals, take up to twenty-five laxatives a day, or engage in violent physical exercise. In extreme cases, to satisfy an overwhelming urge to eat, she may gorge on a quart of ice cream or half a dozen candy bars, and then induce vomiting once again.

The American Digestive Disease Society believes there is a growing percentage of anorectics in the older population as well. In this age group, laxative abuse and deliberate vomiting are practiced by adults as a way to control their weight and "look thin."

Anorexia nervosa, also known as the gorging-purging syndrome, was considered a form of willful starvation when it was first described by Sir William Gull in 1874 in a London medical journal. Today it is recognized as an extremely complex disorder with psychological and physical manifestations. The causes, however, remain a mystery.

Some early psychoanalysts believed that female anorectic patients suffered from the fantasy that they could become pregnant from eating food. Contemporary observers believe that the anorectic fears her developing femininity and refuses to take care of her body and its appetites. A more recent theory holds that anorexia nervosa is a disorder of the hypothalamus, the part of the brain that regulates body temperature, sleep, and food intake. The more disordered the body becomes, the less it seems to be able to recover. Both family stress and the value that this culture places on the underfed "model" look have been implicated as precipitating causes of anorexia nervosa.

The disease can persist for several years. It is extremely difficult to treat because its victims tend to deny that they are ill. Up to fifteen percent of anorectics die from suicide, malnutrition, or other causes doctors cannot identify, even at autopsy. Treatment has ranged from forced feeding to prolonged hospitalization and drugs. In recent years, psychotherapy involving the entire family, behavior modification techniques, and group therapy with other anorectics have been more successful methods of treatment.

Before treatment can begin, however, you must first recognize the symptoms of anorexia nervosa:

- Abnormal weight loss.
- Refusal to eat all but tiny portions of food.
- Excessive exercising.
- Distorted body image (seeing oneself as "fat" when one is actually thin).
- Self-induced vomiting.
- Abuse of laxatives and diet pills to lose weight.
- Depression.
- Binge eating.
- Lack of menstruation.

If a teenager has these symptoms, she / he should be persuaded to see a doctor. Further information and help is available from the National Association of Anorexia Nervosa and Eating Disorders, Inc. (see Appendix A).

CHAPTER 6

Looking Out for Number Two

How Much is Enough?

He used to brew dried senna leaves in a saucepan, and that, along with the suppository melting invisibly in his rectum, comprised *his* witchcraft. . . . As a little boy I sometimes sat in the kitchen and waited with him. But the miracle never came. . . . I remember that when they announced over the radio the explosion of the first atom bomb, he said aloud, 'Maybe that would do the job.' But all catharses were in vain . . .

> — Philip Roth, *Portnoy's Complaint* (N.Y.: Random House, 1967)

HENCE THE AILMENT about which Portnoy's father complained and Abe Lincoln did not, even though our sixteenth president reportedly had only one bowel movement per week. Was Lincoln constipated? Most people would say so, but it didn't seem to bother him.

Four bowel movements a day can be normal and so can one a week. According to the National Center for Health Statistics, 3.8 million people reported in 1979 that they suffered from frequent constipation. Yet many people think they are constipated when they really are not. Constipation is a problem *not* when your bowels fail to move, but when you feel mild pain and discomfort *because* your bowels have not moved. Indeed, "constipation" may be no problem at all, but the ultimate expression of individuality. Martin Luther, founder of the Protestant Reformation, seemed to equate bowel function with rebellious self-expression. "The only portion of the human anatomy which the Pope has had to leave uncontrolled," he once said, "is the hind end."

When constipation occurs, it is caused, above all, by diets that are low in fiber. Fiber or roughage is the nondigestible material found in whole grains, bran, potatoes, cereals, nuts, berries, fresh fruits, and vegetables. As fiber passes through the intestines, basically unchanged by digestion, it absorbs moisture and makes stools larger, softer, and more frequent. Although its true effect on the digestive system is still not established, fiber is thought to have a cleansing function: it dilutes and removes potentially harmful chemicals from the colon. In contrast, it is thought that small stools — which result from low-fiber diets consisting of white bread, sugar, dairy products, meats, fats, and processed foods that have the fiber content removed — cause the colon to work harder and take longer to push the contents along. For example, astronauts on early space flights who were fed nearly fiber-free chemical diets developed constipation that sometimes lasted five to six days.

Vegetables and fruits have been mainstays of the human diet since the time of earliest man. Only recently — in the last fifty to one hundred years — have the United States and other affluent, highly industrialized countries switched to low-fiber diets. Only in recent decades have there been high rates of cancer, heart disease, stroke, and a variety of digestive diseases from hiatus hernia to cancer of the colon.

If your diet is full of fiber and you're *still* constipated, consider: are you depressed? tense? nervous? Feelings like these can cause constipation. You may feel so low that you can't bring yourself to produce anything, not even a stool. This gut reaction goes back to toilet-training days when, on parental command, you had to create something from your own body. Some children, as mentioned earlier, will not release a stool for fear of losing an essential part of their bodies. Others hold back because they are taught that feces are dirty and disgusting. These childhood attitudes may survive — unrecognized — in the constipated adult whose body is still expressing the subconscious feeling, "No, no, I won't go!"

Current theories advocate that parents should not begin toilet training their children too early, nor make a big issue of it. Toilet training begun too early can lead to constipation not only in childhood, but throughout a lifetime.

Like many people who have become constipated under emotional pressure, Thomas Jefferson developed a severe bowel stoppage when he learned that a close friend had defaulted on a loan that Jefferson had cosigned. Robespierre suffered constipation, among other digestive upsets, when his associates gave him a gory description of death on the guillotine. Mahatma Gandhi, who tried to curb his appetite for food and sex, curbed his bowels as well and suffered from constipation. He tried dietary remedies to no avail, and became obsessed with his quest for a cure. Finally, he found relief by applying a poultice of clean, moist earth to his abdomen overnight. George Gershwin had chronic constipation, which he called "composer's stomach." And the novelist Henry James was cursed with constipation during his frequent transcontinental train trips. In one contemporary case, a young woman was constipated for thirteen years, dating back to the day she was fired from a job. She never told anybody about the firing until, thirteen years later, she let out her secret to a psychotherapist. From that day forward, her constipation was cured.

Other causes of constipation include modesty ("If I leave the meeting now, everybody will know where I'm going!"), neglect ("Can't go now — gotta catch bus!"), lack of exercise (a lazy bowel in a lazy body), skipping breakfast (the meal most likely to activate the gastrocolic reflex that in turn activates a bowel movement), and not drinking enough water (which causes stool dehydration and constipation). Even a high toilet seat can cause constipation. A lower seat can make it easier to exert abdominal pressure, hovering high over a public toilet seat can cause the urge — but not the stool — to pass.

You are also likely to become constipated if:

♦ You go on a diet (less food, less stool).

♦ You start eating highly refined foods.

♦ You suddenly stop taking a customary daily glass of prune juice.

♦ You have a bad back, menstrual cramps, or other abdominal pain that makes squeezing down hurt.

♦ You take certain drugs like antacids or opiates.

♦ You have a laxative habit, which also causes diarrhea and an endless cycle of bowel imbalance that will be discussed later in this chapter.

Now that you know the cause of your constipation, you might wonder whether it's serious. As long as you are comfortable and can pass even a hard, dry stool easily, it doesn't matter how often that stool passes. You may have a problem, however, if constipation occurs suddenly or is accompanied by:

♦ Severe abdominal cramps and bloating.

♦ The sudden appearance of very thin, pencil-like or ribbonlike stools.

♦ Pitch black stools or the passage of blood. (Pitch black stools are no cause for concern, however, if you're taking Pepto Bismol or other medications containing iron or bismuth. They tend to turn stools black).

It is as important to know when constipation is *not* a problem, as to know when it is. The national hang-up about constipation, perpetuated in modern times by ads for laxatives, was first articulated and reinforced by John Harvey Kellogg. This late-nineteenth-century "health reformer" and perpetrator of the myth of the daily bowel movement invented a popular line of breakfast cereals that he believed would stamp out sexual feelings, crusaded against clogged colons, and created confusions about bowel function that persist to this day.

Kellogg wrote books, ran spas, and preached the dangers of "autointoxication," the now discredited belief that a missed bowel movement or two means that the toxic contents of the bowel — "a veritable Pandora's box of disease" as Kellogg described them — are absorbed by the rest of the body. Kellogg's way of averting this "disaster" was to sweep the colon clean of all body wastes and food residues.

For most people, he proclaimed, it takes about forty hours to clear food residues from the last two feet of the colon, or about twenty times longer than it should. Hence, he devised eighteen rules for unclogging the colon, some — though certainly not all — of which are accepted in medical practice today. For example, he recommended eating several ounces of fiber daily in the form of bran, green vegetables, and whole grains. He urged that meals be regular. Exercise, he realized, promotes bowel action, and laxative drugs do great harm. He also recognized that the squatting position is a great aid to bowel movements. He then went on to declare that the bowels must move at least three times daily, at the exact same hour, if possible. Not only should the bowels move, but the colon should be cleaned out as well. To insure this outcome, he recommended a warm enema totaling about three pints of water after each bowel movement. A cold morning bath, he said, might aid bowel action, but if that didn't work, he recommended massaging the colon, vibrating the abdomen, and, in particularly costive (stubbornly constipated) cases, applying electricity to the abdominal muscles, rectum, and colon.

In later years, his advice became even more elaborate:

♦ Answer the "call," even the slightest, at once. Delays of five or ten minutes may be disastrous.
♦ Give the bowels a chance to evacuate on rising, at bedtime, and after each meal, even if there is no "call."
♦ Take a two-quart enema in the evening, and then take another half-pint of warm water to be retained overnight.

By the turn of the century, the bowel was coming into its own. To thousands of spa clients — mostly tired businessmen suffering from dyspepsia — Kellogg prescribed purifying diets from above, two daily enemas from below, and treatment with an enema machine that could shoot fifteen gallons of water through the bowels in minutes. Kellogg fed patients with high blood pressure ten to fourteen pounds of grapes daily; others were given half a pint of milk every half-hour, supplemented by fruit twice daily and three table-spoons of paraffin oil four times a day. In one treatment, patients were rubbed while in the nude with a paste of salt and water, then subjected to electrical stinging and tickling of the skin. The treatments must have had some appeal: Kellogg's patients included some of the wealthiest and most powerful people in the country. Kellogg's spa attendants also offered stomach irrigation, bladder irrigation, vaginal irrigation (administered on a special marble-covered couch that wouldn't get a lady's clothes wet), uterine irrigation, and rectal irrigation.

Water, Water Everywhere

Enemas have a long history. The ancient Egyptians — inspired by the ibis, which supposedly used its curved beak to inject sea water into its rectum — used to purge themselves on three successive days each month. They retained enemas overnight for medicinal purposes. Nutrient enemas were also given in an attempt to reach the stomach, south to north. Ancient physicians mistakenly believed the stomach could gradually draw upward any nourishment present in the lower bowel. Thus, physicians would clean the colon and inject a nutrient enema of milk, broth, eggs, or gruel.

Tobacco-smoke enemas were a popular way to stimulate the intestine. They were administered with an iron or brass capsule large enough to hold about half an ounce of tobacco. To this capsule were fastened two tubes, one for insertion into the anus, and the other for insertion into the mouth of an assistant who would blow through it and force the tobacco smoke in the capsule through the tube into the anus.

In the seventeenth century, holy water enemas were reported to have successfully exorcised devils from possessed nuns, and in late-seventeenth-century France, clysters became a social fad. Although "clyster" means washing out or douching, and enema means to throw in or inject, the words have been used to mean the same thing. Louis XIII reportedly took 220 enemas during the last six months of his life, and even had them given to his dogs when they were ill. Ladies of the French court took several enemas daily to keep their skin white and complexions fresh. Ladies-in-waiting administered clysters to the Duchess of Burgundy so skillfully that the courtiers at her salon in Versailles hardly noticed it. Soon, the common people began following the royal suit, and the daily enema became a ritual akin to brushing the teeth.

Voltaire, the eighteenth-century author and philosopher, was so despondent one time that he told a friend he had decided to hang himself. The friend called the next day, anxious to know whether Voltaire was alive and well, and was delighted to find that the great man had undergone a complete change of mood overnight. Voltaire met him with a smile and an explanation: "I have been well washed out!"

To meet the demand, many new kinds of enema apparatus were designed to supplement the early reeds, funnels, and gourds. The piston syringe made its debut sometime during the fifteenth century. In uppercrust France, the syringe was made of porcelain, gilded silver, and mother-of-pearl. Some models were designed so that they could be used in the sitting position; others, so that piston pressure could be applied from a wall or bedpost. Both models posed dangers of perforating the intestine if inserted carelessly.

The next important development in enema technology was John Read's invention in the early nineteenth century of the two-way syringe with ball valves. It could be used to blow smoke into the rectum, draw milk from a breast, and water roses. It was a most useful and imitated machine. Next to appear was a rather villainous mechanical irrigator invented by the Frenchman Maurice Eguisier in 1848. The piston was controlled by a cylinder spring that, once released, caused the piston to expel the fluid with considerable power — too much power for the tender tissues of the bowel. About the same time, Alfred Higginson, a Liverpool surgeon, was busy inventing the "English syringe," which incorporated an ingenious system of valves that forced any quantity of water in under pressure.

Meanwhile, the forerunner of the modern collapsible rubber enema bag had emerged from the Amazon, where the native Amerindians had developed a simple rubber bag with a conical nozzle. Into these bags, syringes, and funnels have been poured all sorts of mixtures, from hemp, honey, herbs, and human milk, to soap, molasses, lemon juice, and glycerine.

Enemas are currently undergoing somewhat of a revival in a modern day "colonics" craze. Amid ads promising to rid the body of impurities, readjust the diet, and even cure cancer, chiropractors, nutritional counselors, and colonic parlors are charging money for a service that will eventually shut down the natural functioning of the bowel reflex and will virtually destroy the bowel. Many people take enemas almost every day for decades. Two women who had taken daily enemas for forty years finally had to undergo complete removal of their large intestines because their bowels would no longer function. The surgery involved attachment of the far end of the small intestine to the abdominal wall so that waste products could be collected in a bag.

In another instance, seven people died after receiving colonic irrigation — a series of machine-administered enemas to "wash out" the colon. The deaths were caused by amebiasis, an intestinal infection usually transmitted by mouth but, in this case, transmitted by the use of improperly disinfected machines.

Several other people have died from a cancer treatment consisting of a natural food diet and coffee enemas administered every two hours. One forty-six-year-old woman died after receiving about a dozen coffee enemas in one night, which added up to three or four per hour. Physicians describing the case in a medical journal said death probably resulted from potassium depletion and fluid overload. Actor Steve McQueen was receiving coffee enemas in a Mexican health clinic shortly before his death from cancer. A young woman who took coffee enemas for years without any problem once told a friend about her predilection. The friend asked, "Do you take cream?"

There is no doubt that enemas have a pleasurable side. As J.P. Donleavy notes in *The Unexpurgated Code,* ". . . there are far worse ways to spend a half an hour . . . a penile erection at this time is regarded as an unavoidable reaction to internal water pressures and no apologies are necessary." A poem published in *Knickerbocker* in the mid-1800s does not seem out-of-date:

> It's water, water everywhere,
> And quarts to drink if you can bear;
> 'Tis well that we are made of clay
> For common dust would wash away!

There are legitimate medical uses for enemas, especially in diagnosis and detection of colon cancer, when a thorough, cleansing enema can literally mean the difference between life and death. Of the five to fifteen percent of cancers of the colon that are missed during barium X ray examination, seventy-five percent are mistaken for or hidden by fecal material because of poor preparation of the colon by enema. The unnecessary delay this causes in early treatment could cost you your life.

Rough Remedies

The nationwide urge to eliminate feces is expressed in other ways as well. Constipation "therapies" in the past have included hypnosis, abdominal massage, forced dilation of the anus, and electrical stimulation with alternating current, known as faradism. In this treatment, two plate electrodes measuring about four by five inches, are placed on either side of the abdomen. Then an electric current of thirty milliamperes is turned on for ten minutes, causing contraction of the abdominal muscles. A related treatment, faradization of the rectum, is performed with a rectal electrode and a six-inch soft rectal tube with an opening for filling the rectum with fluid. After 1½ ounces of lukewarm saline solution is injected, a second electrode is passed over the abdomen along the path of the large intestine. This causes the abdominal wall to contract, and the patient to feel a pronounced prickling in the rectum.

People tolerated these rough remedies because they were sold on the dangers of constipation. Straining at stool, many people believed, could lead to eye and brain hemorrhage, not to mention malaria, nocturnal emissions, and excessive sexual indulgence.

Perhaps the most radical remedy of all was practiced by Sir William Arbuthnot Lane who advocated, as a treatment for what he called "chronic intestinal stasis" (constipation), surgical removal of the colon. He performed at least a thousand of these operations from 1903 until his death in 1938, and justified them on the basis that fecal bacteria shorten life.

Laxatives are the modern rough remedy for constipation. Doctors do not know exactly how they work, but they do know that laxatives cause more constipation than they cure. Ever since the days of Beecham's Pills and Eno's Fruit Salts, constipation has become increasingly commercialized. Indeed, some of the leading drug houses were founded on such products. What the commercials do not tell you is that laxatives, like enemas, can damage the bowel reflex. Furthermore, laxatives are irritants, can be habit forming, and can interfere with other digestive processes.

Laxatives create the problem they were meant to cure. People who get "hooked" on these drugs, and engage in long-term, frequently hidden overindulgence, often lead lives of chronic ill health. Doctors are hard pressed to prove a patient is abusing laxatives and sometimes, as a last resort, must search their patients' possessions for laxatives before a successful confrontation is possible. The patient may have undergone many expensive hospitalizations and surgical procedures before this happens. Many people who abuse laxatives are unable to give them up even when their habit is discovered.

Among the current over-the-counter drugs for constipation, some are safe, some are not. Mineral oil should not be used with other laxatives, and should not be used very often because it impairs absorption of vitamins A, D, and E.

Laxatives like milk of magnesia are dangerous to people with kidney disease because they cause the body to retain harmful amounts of magnesium.

Loosening Up

Constipation is rarely a symptom of disease, and you seldom need a doctor or drugs to treat it. Usually, all you need to do is:

◆ Eat a high-fiber diet, the foremost remedy for constipation.

◆ Take a "daily constitutional," or start swimming, bicycling, or engaging in some other activity.

◆ Exercise to strengthen your abdominal muscles so they can place pressure on a sluggish gut.

◆ If diet and exercise don't work, try a bulk laxative such as Metamucil or Effersylium.

◆ Drink lots of fluids: eight to ten full glasses daily, including prune juice, which contains a chemical that gets the gut moving.

◆ Eat breakfast, also to get things moving.

◆ Drink a cup of coffee or something warm to stimulate the gastrocolic reflex.

◆ Lower your toilet seat.

It is said that the ideal posture for defecation is the squatting position, which allows your thighs to press against the abdominal muscles and increase the pressure inside your abdomen. Some advocates of squatting even suggest that you squat atop the seat of a conventional toilet. The high seat was an unfortunate design feature of the flush toilet. That design, in turn, was probably inspired by the portable thrones called "close stools" that English and French monarchs employed to set themselves off from the common folk who squatted.

Whether you sit or squat, consider this final remedy for constipation: Immanuel Kant, the German philosopher, thought that laughter benefits the intestinal tract. Is laughter also a cure for constipation? If so, a good joke book might be part of your home pharmacy.

CHAPTER 7

What Makes Sammy Run?

THE IRREVERENT ANSWER would be the green apple quick-step, Montezuma's revenge, or Delhi belly. But for people who have the kind of diarrhea that attacks without warning and sends them to the bathroom six to twenty-four times a day, diarrhea is no joke.

Diarrhea ranges from occasional loose stools and cramps (which, strictly speaking, do not qualify as diarrhea), to the profuse, watery diarrhea caused by gastroenteritis, to the kind that strikes infants, to the kind that strikes travelers, to the kind that is sexually transmitted. Aretaeus of Cappadocia, an ancient Greek physician, defined diarrhea as "the discharge of undigested food in a fluid state . . . no part of the digestive process having been properly done, except the commencement." A modern Mayo Clinic physician says it this way: "When the sequence comprising integrated intestinal function fails, fecal excretion is inconvenient, bulky and liquid."

◊   ◊   ◊

The Enemy Below

For years, doctors thought that diarrhea was caused by increased activity of the intestine. Recently, this thinking changed when researchers noticed that some of the viruses and bacteria that invade the bowel can multiply and produce toxins that irritate the bowel and make it weep, or pour fluid into the stool, thereby causing cramping, abdominal pain, and diarrhea. There are other mechanisms that cause diarrhea. For example, if diarrhea is triggered by the gastrocolic reflex (see Chapter 1), it can occur within five minutes after overeating sets off waves of peristalsis throughout your intestinal tract. What comes out, of course, is food you ate several days earlier. Diarrhea caused by a virus or bacteria, on the other hand, can take hours or days to develop, depending on which agent is involved, how much of it you have consumed, and how long it takes to multiply and produce toxins as it travels from mouth to anus.

Thus, diarrhea is nature's way of protecting you against potentially poisonous material by getting rid of these bacteria and their toxins. It's a comforting thought, but one that people lunging for the loo seldom savor. Thus, the intestinal tract serves not only as an organ of digestion, but as an organ of defense. The sea cucumber protects itself by getting rid of its entire intestinal tract and growing a new one whenever it is disturbed. Higher animals have developed more complex systems for selecting food, but their intestinal defense mechanisms remain primitive.

Nearly everybody has urgent calls to stool from time to time. According to the Metropolitan Life Insurance Company, diarrhea is one of the leading causes of absence from work, especially among women. It accounted for fourteen percent of all hospital admissions of United States troops serving in the Vietnam War, and throughout the world, it is the leading killer of infants and children.

The enemy below could also be a parasite, physical disease such as diabetes or uremia, bowel obstruction, antibiotic, laxative habit, food allergies, or improper digestion of food in the small intestine. Diarrhea often occurs before the onset of a woman's menstrual period because menstruation normally alters the fluid balance of the body, causing it to retain water. This, in turn, leads to increased motor activity in the intestines — and to diarrhea.

Even diet mints can cause diarrhea. Two physicians wrote a letter to the *Journal of the American Medical Association* telling how one of them had eaten twelve diet mints during a two-hour medical meeting. Thirty minutes after consuming the last mint, he developed cramps, gas, and diarrhea. Only when a further episode required hospitalization did he read the label and discover that the artificial sweetener was sorbitol, a nondigestible sugar alcohol which sits in the intestine and is fermented by bacteria. Far more sorbitol than saccharin is needed to sweeten food, and sorbitol, taken in quantity, can upset the stomach and intestine. Even with smaller quantities, upsets can occur. Sorbitol is a common ingredient in medicinal syrups and gelatin capsules; foods, gums, and candies for diabetics and dieters; and certain toothpastes (it makes them taste better). So if abdominal symptoms occur after you've used any of these products, check to see if sorbitol is to blame.

Another cause of diarrhea is Chinese restaurant syndrome or CRS II (see Chapter 4 for a description of CRS I). CRS II causes nausea, stomach cramps, and dehydration. It strikes from one to twenty-four hours after eating Chinese food, and lasts about a day. The culprit in this case is not monosodium glutamate (MSG), but spores of the *Bacillus cereus* organism. Fried rice is the apparent vehicle for this bacteria. When boiled rice is left out of the refrigerator, as Chinese restaurant chefs commonly do to keep it from clumping, *B. cereus* spores found in uncooked rice may survive and grow. Flash frying or rewarming just before serving the rice does not destroy the toxin. Fortunately, CRS II is fairly mild, and seldom needs a doctor's care.

B. cereus has caused food poisoning outbreaks in the United States and Europe by contaminating meat, vegetables, milk, and cocoa. The organism has also been found in seasoning mixes, spices, dry potatoes, minced meat, puddings, and spaghetti sauces—places you would not expect to find toxins lurking. *B. cereus* can also be transmitted person-to-person. The most common bacterial causes of diarrhea in the United States are *Campylobacter* and *Shigella*. The former is transmitted in water or by direct contamination, and the latter, by person-to-person contact and, occasionally, in food. Bacteria that infect food include *Salmonella* (commonly found in poultry and eggs) and *Escherichia coli*. They have different incubation periods. For example, *Salmonella* may take eight to forty-eight hours to incubate and cause diarrhea, while *Campylobacter* may take two to ten days. Even public health experts find it difficult to determine which organisms have caused food poisoning outbreaks involving dozens or hundreds of people. In general, if you are exposed to contaminated food and, soon after, suffer from vomiting and diarrhea, you probably have food poisoning.

It was only recently discovered that diarrhea can also be sexually transmitted by oral-anal contact. For example, seventy to ninety percent of all of San Francisco's reported cases of shigellosis and amebiasis — severe infections of the intestinal tract — occur in the sexually active male homosexual community. In the gay community of New York City's Lower West Side, the carrier rate for these pathogens is twenty-five percent, compared to three percent in another community that usually had a high rate of such infections. This problem, known as the "gay bowel syndrome," may be a misnomer since enteric infections also occur among heterosexual men and women who have oral-anal contact or anal intercourse.

Diarrhea is also a body reaction to short-term stress or long-term psychological problems. The normal motion of the bowels speeds up, sometimes within minutes of eating, and causes food to rush through, triggering the cramps that usually accompany diarrhea.

"Nervous diarrhea," or the "shits," is a fear reaction experienced by athletes, soldiers in battle, lawyers preparing to speak to juries, and journalists facing deadlines. Nervous diarrhea often accompanies sexual or marital discord; conflict with teachers, bosses, and coworkers; unexpressed anxieties about losing your job; or fear of failing an examination at school. Emotionally-induced diarrhea tends to strike meticulous and conscientious people who are highly sensitive, who depend upon others for decision-making and emotional support, and who harbor deep feelings of guilt.

Many people afflicted with persistent diarrhea face situational demands they feel they cannot meet, or are under stresses of which they are unaware. A newlywed woman, for example, suffered from after-dinner diarrhea throughout the first year of her marriage. She worked all day and was expected to come home every night to cook a full meal and clean up afterwards. Her protest was expressed through her gut rather than in words, and the diarrhea did not stop until the twin stress of working and keeping house came to an end.

The eminent gastroenterologist Dr. Franz J. Ingelfinger once described a form of nervous diarrhea known as "the morning rush syndrome." He described it as a series of urgent bowel movements, with or without cramps, that begin when one first gets up in the morning. Each movement would prove more watery than the preceding, until the diarrhea ran out, as it were, by midmorning.

One patient had a series of diarrhea attacks one hour after her evening meal, and at no other time. Six patients with nervous diarrhea stated that their symptoms improved dramatically during holidays and worsened during emotional upsets. The respected psychoanalyst Franz Alexander, who wrote some of the earliest works on gastroemotional problems in the mid-1930s, once noted that people who develop diarrhea may have a fundamental desire to give or eliminate, while people with constipation want to hold back or retain.

Laxative abuse is another cause of diarrhea that may be hard to cure, since most laxative abusers refuse to acknowledge their habit, even though they are having a dozen or more loose, watery stools per day. Deep down, they might believe that the contents of their intestines are dirty or dangerous — something to be gotten rid of. Often, even after extensive physical examination and laboratory tests reveal no organic or structural reasons for the diarrhea, these individuals still deny their habit. In one extreme case, a patient finally admitted he had taken twelve chocolate laxatives, several tablespoonsful of milk of magnesia, and other laxative preparations every day for the previous four years. He did it to get attention and sympathy from his family: he felt they were ignoring him. Rather than give up his habit, he later underwent several hospitalizations and three abdominal surgeries to repair laxative damage to his intestines. Often, when no other proof of laxative abuse can be found, a physician will examine the mucous membrane of the colon through a proctoscope, or tube inserted into the rectum. A dark brown or black mucosal lining is a sign of laxative abuse.

"Stomach Flu"

One of the most common causes of diarrhea is "stomach flu," an acute viral infection of the digestive system, otherwise known as intestinal flu, or twenty-four-hour grippe. Second only to the common cold as a cause of illness in the United States, this is a self-limited form of gastroenteritis that causes fever, chills, stomach ache, nausea, abdominal cramps, and diarrhea, in varying combinations. Stomach flu lasts one or two days, is rarely serious, and can be treated with bed rest and clear liquids to replace lost fluids and salts. Only when vomiting and diarrhea are very severe or last longer than twenty-four hours in adults is it necessary to call a doctor.

If stomach flu occurs in infants, dehydration is a more serious threat, and you should call a physician immediately. This form of gastroenteritis is one of the five leading causes of childhood death in the United States. About five years ago, a tiny wheel-shaped virus was identified as the leading cause of diarrhea in infants and young children throughout the world. Called the "rotavirus" because of its roundness, this organism has caused winter epidemics of diarrhea in the world's largest cities, including New York, and year-round epidemics in tropical regions. Rotavirus diarrhea causes an estimated five to ten million deaths annually, mostly of children (see Chapter 12). Researchers have discovered that the virus strikes virtually every young person in this country by late childhood. It affects not only children, but, in many cases, their parents and other family members as well. Scientists at the National Institutes of Health have developed a technique for growing many strains of rotavirus in the laboratory, bringing the world one step closer to developing an effective vaccine to prevent this disease.

Turista!

Bacteria — especially the colonic bacteria *Escherichia coli* — cause a more severe form of diarrhea than viruses do. Normally, you harbor these microbes in your intestines, but when you travel, you may pick up one of a tremendous number of alien strains that populate the earth. They find their way into food and water and from there, into the intestinal tract. These microbes cause an estimated sixty to ninety percent of traveler's diarrhea, forcing many a traveler to spend vacation hours studying tiles from a seated position. If enough alien *E. coli* populate the intestine, they produce a toxin which injures the intestinal wall, interferes with normal absorption, and results in watery stools, fever, and cramps. In addition, *E. coli* cause the intestine to actively secrete fluid, which makes the diarrhea-wracked body even less able to absorb food and nutrients into the blood stream.

Another important cause of traveler's diarrhea is the intestinal parasite *Giardia lamblia*. It also causes an intestinal disease called giardiasis. Although many people carry *G. lamblia* around in their guts without ill effect, the problem comes when you get an overdose from drinking unsafe water. This can happen abroad or, as one recent outbreak proves, in Aspen, Colorado. Even ice cubes in the drink served in that quaint foreign café, the lettuce and fruit in your salad, and the water you use to brush your teeth can send you into paroxysms of cramps and diarrhea.

Boiling water with an electric immersion coil, or treating it with water purification tablets will protect you from that source of infection. You also should avoid milk and milk products, including frozen confections sold by street venders, because freezing may preserve, not destroy, bacteria. Avoid poolside smorgasbords or buffets that are so popular in the tropics, and when swimming, try not to swallow or get water in your mouth. The water in most American- and

European-run hotels overseas is usually safe, but to be sure, check with a travel agent, airline, or a good guide book.

Travelers from underdeveloped countries sometimes get traveler's diarrhea, but usually less severely than travelers, say, from Canada. If the former succumb to the "bug" in New York City, for example, they can call it "Bronx Belly" or "Rockefeller's Revenge."

These days, when you travel, the advice "Don't drink the water, don't eat the food," may not be enough to prevent the intestinal agonies of the European Grand Tour. You also should know that the stresses of altered eating habits, strange food, jet lag, tension, excitement, and decreased oxygen aboard airplanes all contribute to traveler's syndrome.

Consider the stresses of travel, from prevacation jitters to postvacation blues, when you return from a vacation wishing you could take a vacation. The stresses include guilt (because, after all, you don't really deserve a vacation), unmet expectations, disrupted routine, and logistical pressures of stopping the mail, kenneling the cat, and footing the bill for the trip. Another stress may be the unavoidable closeness to children and spouse who are kept at an emotional distance the rest of the year. Such feelings may persuade you to avoid vacations altogether, develop fear of flying, get sick during the trip, or resort to some other subconscious sabotage.

The true nature of traveler's syndrome was explored several years ago by the American Digestive Disease Society (ADDS), which sent a questionnaire to readers of a newsletter called *Travel Advisor*. The questionnaire asked about lifestyles, food preferences, personality types, and digestive problems while traveling. Although the survey did not settle the question of whether tension ranks with contaminated water and food as a cause of "turista," it did reveal that seventy-two percent of the participants had digestive problems during their vacations, and that eighty-seven percent had upsets that lasted from two to seven days after they returned home.

One commercial airline pilot who had flown for ten years to Asia, Central and South America, the Mediterranean, and the Caribbean (turista territories all) reported in an ADDS newsletter, *Living Healthy:*

I have come to the conclusion that the vast majority of stomach and intestinal problems are the result of two factors; being convinced that one is going to have a problem and the attempt on the part of most Americans to seek out and obtain U.S. foods in foreign parts. A hamburger, hot dog, fried chicken or chicken-salad sandwich in many countries could turn out to be most anything . . .

The same pilot became accustomed to food and beverages in the countries along his route, although, he reported, "I do tend to temper [the water] with 'medicinal' Scotch . . ." You can learn to tolerate alien strains of *E. coli* through continuous mild exposure. However, immunity also depends on the number and strength of the bacteria. In places where sanitation is good and you encounter relatively few bacteria, diarrhea will tend to be mild. In the tropics, where *E. coli* are more virulent and plentiful, watch out.

Several women who usually traveled with their husbands described the tensions of traveling alone, and of having to fend for themselves in strange surroundings. Others cited the pressures of compulsory traveling for business and official purposes. As one respondent said, "I would bet that by far the largest number of gastric and intestinal sufferers like myself are rendered that way by the foreknowledge . . . that if you don't want to lose money in business, you've got to endure the Italian plumbing, the traumatic Slav parties, and Heathrow Airport . . ." The president of a travel agency offered these survival strategies in the same issue of *Living Healthy:*

- ◆ Learn as much as possible about the place you will be visiting to relieve apprehension about a new environment.
- ◆ Learn about food and water safety in the places you will visit.
- ◆ Learn in advance where to go for medical and other emergencies.
- ◆ Break out of your daily routine about a week before you travel, especially your eating and sleeping patterns.
- ◆ While abroad, don't get run down and don't go on eating binges.

An additional precaution, suggested in the February 1979 issue of *Travel and Holiday* magazine, is frequent and thorough handwashing. The *E. coli* bacteria that cause so much traveler's diarrhea lurk everywhere, including your body. Many travelers peel their oranges with contaminated hands, and wonder why they get turista! In fact, handwashing will help prevent the transmission of all kinds of infections.

An unusual case of traveler's diarrhea occurred during a cavalry hike in 1936 from Ft. Sheridan, Illinois to Grand Rapids, Michigan. An entire cavalry company, including the horses, contracted diarrhea from contaminated water. Army doctors put the men (not the horses) on mashed banana, grated raw apple, and cooled boiled milk. One survivor told his wife, "Don't stand there and gloat just because you're comfortably constipated!"

Cures, Cures, Cures

Thousands of remedies have been tried for traveler's diarrhea. Many do not work at all; others work, but should not be used on a regular basis. Kaopectate may help in mild cases of diarrhea. Medications such as Lomotil or preparations that contain paregoric are stronger. Lomotil provides temporary relief of cramps and diarrhea by slowing down the action of the digestive tract, but does not address the cause of the problem and, in some cases, prolongs it. For example, when diarrhea is caused by *Salmonella* or *Shigella*, Lomotil can cause the body to retain these organisms and their toxins. Sometimes travelers take Lomotil almost indiscriminately to calm their rampaging intestines. One tourist who believed in being prepared was caught in a vicious cycle when he overdosed with paregoric, which geared down his gut so much he became constipated. He then reached for remedies to loosen his bowels, only to find that again he had diarrhea! Furthermore, if taken over a long period of time, Lomotil leads to drug dependency because it causes the colon to lose its tone. In extreme cases, this drug can cause the diarrhea it is meant to cure because it essentially paralyzes the gut, a condition doctors call "lead pipe" colon.

The antibiotic doxycycline — taken two days prior to and throughout the trip — reduces the incidence and severity of traveler's diarrhea caused by *E. coli*. But the drug has not been recommended for prolonged periods because *E. coli* tend quickly to become resistant to antibiotics. Another problem is that doxycycline causes side effects in some persons, including oversensitivity to sunlight and gastrointestinal upset!

Another remedy for traveler's diarrhea is Pepto Bismol. In early 1980, the *Journal of the American Medical Association (JAMA)* reported that when subsalicylate bismuth — the active ingredient in Pepto Bismol that also helps relieve upset stomach, indigestion, and nausea — was tested in a group of American students spending the summer in Guadalajara, Mexico, the occurrence and severity of diarrhea was reduced from sixty-one to twenty-three percent. The longer Pepto Bismol was used, moreover, the more effective it became. Unfortunately, the amount of Pepto Bismol that was taken in the study was 240 milliliters, or one eight-ounce bottle daily. Thus, a three-week stay for two people would require forty-two 8-ounce bottles of Pepto Bismol, no light load. As the *JAMA* article noted, "Even if these medications could be accommodated in a forty-four-pound weight allotment, many tourists might be reluctant to face this drug four times a day during what should be a vacation." It is not yet known whether a lesser amount would be effective. In addition, Pepto Bismol might produce constipation in older persons, although the young students in the study were not so affected. Finally, not only is the dosage large, but, according to the study, about twenty-five percent of everybody who takes Pepto Bismol would not be helped anyway. Despite these disadvantages, the Pepto Bismol approach avoids the unpleasant side effects of antibiotics, and is a safe treatment that could help many a beleaguered traveler.

Recent studies in Central America, sponsored by the National Institutes of Health, show that certain drugs such as Enterovioform, which were once widely used to treat traveler's diarrhea, are not only ineffective, but may actually make the condition worse. Other new treatments under development for traveler's diarrhea include oral vaccines, which are more effective in stimulating immunity in the intestinal tract, and new combinations of antibiotics which have been found to effectively reduce the duration of diarrhea caused by *E. coli.*

In general, if you're down with diarrhea:

◆ Get plenty of physical rest.

◆ Avoid solid foods. Drink warm — never hot — broth and tea, water, flat soda, and other mild liquids to replace fluids and salts lost through diarrhea.

◆ Drink fluids containing sugar and salt, such as Gatorade.

◆ As your condition improves, add soups, Jell-O, applesauce, and bland foods like rice and toast.

◆ Drink liquids between meals rather than with them.

◆ Replace potassium, which is depleted when you have diarrhea, by eating bananas, potatoes, meat, and fish, or ask your doctor about potassium supplements.

◆ Until your intestines calm down, avoid milk and high-fiber foods like fruits and vegetables with seeds and tough skins.

◆ Don't eat foods that are fatty, spicy, or that cause gas or cramps. These include carbonated drinks, beer, beans, cabbage, cauliflower, sweets, and chewing gum

◆ Work up slowly to a normal high-fiber diet.

◆ If a clear liquid diet does not work, try a tablespoon of Kaopectate after each loose bowel movement.

◆ If Kaopectate does not work, try paregoric, a narcotic which slows down the digestive tract. Parapectolin and Parelixir may be available without a prescription.

◆ If your diarrhea lasts longer than seventy-two hours, if it has blood in it, or if you have severe abdominal pain, see a doctor.

You might also try a simple home remedy — a mixture of sugar and table salt — to relieve the dehydration that is an uncomfortable aftermath of diarrhea. Versions of this remedy — known medically as oral glucose / electrolyte solutions — have been used for years to cure the life-threatening massive dehydration of cholera victims in East Pakistan. This remedy, however, is safe only for healthy adults and school-aged children. It is not safe for preschool children or babies, or for adults with heart, kidney, or adrenal gland diseases.

The formula is simple. In one quart of water, mix ½ teaspoon of table salt, ½ teaspoon of baking soda, ¼ teaspoon of potassium chloride, and 2 tablespoons of glucose. The last two ingredients are available in powdered or crystal form in most pharmacies at nominal cost. A physician's prescription may be necessary for the potassium chloride. As long as the dehydrated feeling persists, the more you drink of this mixture, the better. This balanced glucose-salt solution allows such rapid absorption through the intestinal wall that dehydration is overcome.

No commercial preparations of this salt-sugar solution are available in the United States, although several similar solutions are marketed in foreign countries. Gatorade and similar beverages contain different ingredients, and are designed to relieve salt loss due to sweating, although they may help relieve diarrhea-caused dehydration as well.

The salt-sugar solution will relieve dehydration from diarrhea, whether the cause is traveling, food allergies, laxatives, emotional upset, infections, drug reactions, or food poisoning from $100-a-plate dinners. It is also a good remedy for a hangover.

CHAPTER 8

Gone with the Wind

. . . The stomach (crammed from every dish,
A tomb of boiled and roast, and flesh and fish,
Where bile, and wind, and phlegm, and acid jar,
And all the man is one intestine war)
> — Alexander Pope, "Second Book
> of Horace, Satire II"

IT SEEMS THAT the stomach — no matter how often you tell
it to "shut up!" — talks back. When it does, it speaks a gut-
tural language of gas, belching, borborygmi, hiccups, and
halitosis. J.P. Donleavy called these conditions "vilenesses
various" in *The Unexpurgated Code*. You might call them life's
little problems that threaten social conventions far more than
they threaten health.

A large part of the practice of gastroenterology concerns itself with treating vague, ill-defined symptoms of gas-
eous discomfort: bloating, belching, gurgles, growls, and
flatulence. Life's little problems, however, seldom need a
doctor's care. You can usually take care of them yourself,
once you understand that they have causes, cures, and —
inevitably — emotional roots.

◇ ◇ ◇

Gas

"Flatuosities," as Hippocrates called them, were originally thought to originate entirely within the body. Ancient physicians who become known as "pneumatists" named the condition *morbus ructuosus,* and ascribed all sorts of disorders to it. Not until the end of the eighteenth century was the notion of morbus abandoned, and men of science became interested in the actual nature and origin of intestinal gas. Human volunteers were not easy to come by, so scientists examined freshly executed criminals. Still, no precise descriptions of the chemistry of intestinal gas came from the crude methods employed at the time.

During the early nineteenth century, the idea occurred that air swallowing might also cause flatulence. In 1813, the illustrious French physiologist Francois Magendie reported the case of a conscript who practiced auto-inflation in order to avoid military service. Magendie also pointed out that air-swallowing in humans was not unlike "cribbing" (windsucking) in horses, and that the practice was by no means rare. In fact, he found that in eight out of one hundred students examined, it could be self-taught. Only later was it understood that air swallowing is a perfectly normal process, and that some air is swallowed with food, drinks, and saliva. People who eat too fast, smoke, or are emotionally distressed swallow so much air, however, that at some point it causes one of two things: belching or that other socially inadmissible gut reaction from the other end.

The next source of scientific curiosity was the question of how much gas people pass. Researchers in the early 1940s inserted thick-walled rubber balloons attached to colon tubes about ten centimeters up the rectums of five healthy young medical students. The tubes were held in place by adhesive tape so that the volunteers could go about their business each day. The researchers changed the balloons every twelve hours and measured the volume of gas in them. Results showed that the subjects passed about 527 cubic centimeters of gas daily.

Further research established that the normal person

passes four hundred to one thousand cubic centimeters of gas in a day, roughly the volume of one to three cans of beer. The composition of intestinal gas, still other studies have revealed, consists of varying proportions of carbon dioxide, hydrogen, methane, nitrogen, and oxygen. Some individuals have been found to manufacture no intestinal methane at all, while a third of the population generates large amounts.

Next, science turned to causes and confirmed what your ancestors had long ago observed: intestinal gas is closely connected to diet. For some people, milk and milk products are gas-producing. But, more often, the foods at fault include brussels sprouts, cabbage, cauliflower, onions, and beans.

The ancient Romans believed that the souls of the dead reposed in beans. They (the beans) were eaten with respect and ceremony. Today, beans are the food most often blamed for flatulence, and also for musical stomach. They contain peculiar carbohydrates called oligosaccharides, which cannot be digested by the normal intestinal tract. Consequently, they pass into the lower intestine where bacteria cause these carbohydrates to ferment and form carbon dioxide and hydrogen gases.

This does not daunt organic gardeners and beanophiles: "Give beans a chance," they cry aloud and on bumper stickers. "The more you eat, the less you fart." The digestive system, they say, will calm down and the flatulence will subside once beans become a regular diet item.

Medical science has not put this claim to test, but scientists are trying to breed a nonflatugenic, or gasless bean that lacks these oligosaccharides. Already, one study observed that navy bean meal caused 2.52 times as much gas as dehulled, defatted soybean meal. Another study of six bean preparations showed that mature lima beans caused more farting than navy or green lima beans, and twice as much as pork and beans. Pork and beans were as flatugenic as Boston baked beans.

Some of the greatest contributions to public knowledge about flatulence come from Dr. Michael D. Levitt of the University of Minnesota Hospitals, known as the physician who gave class to gas and status to flatus and who, in his own

words, has attempted to "pump some data into a field that
has been filled largely with hot air."

In 1976, Dr. Levitt reported on a twenty-eight-year-old
patient who, for the previous five years, had been gravely
gassy. This patient was passing up to 346 milliliters of gas
per hour, compared to the normal 100. At one point, the
young man passed gas 141 times on one day, including 70
passages in a four-hour period. His performance, a footnote
in a medical journal article pointed out, was pending recog-
nition by the *Guinness Book of World Records*. The high volume of gas occurred when the patient consumed nothing but
milk. But even when his diet did not include milk, he still
had a gas crisis, so he started keeping "flatographic" records
of when he passed gas and what he had eaten in an attempt
to develop a flatus-free, palatable diet. As Dr. Levitt noted in
a 1976 article in the *New England Journal of Medicine*, his
patient was testing a variety of foods, "thus far without even
a whiff of success."

In 1979, another article appeared by Dr. Levitt and his
patient, under the nom de plume of L.O. Sutalf (read it back-
wards). They reported that Dr. Levitt's earlier observation
had been premature, and Mr. Sutalf had since discovered a
diet which left him "normo-flatulent." Over a two-year period, Mr. Sutalf had tested 130 different foods, noting each
day which foods he ate, when he passed gas, and whether
the amount he passed was small ("a squeaker") or apprecia-
ble.

According to this unprecedented account of a low-flatus
diet, the foods that produced "normal" levels of flatulence
for Mr. Sultalf include:

- ◆ Meat, fowl, and fish.
- ◆ Vegetables — lettuce, cucumber, broccoli, peppers,
avocado, cauliflower, tomato, asparagus, zucchini, okra,
and olives.
- ◆ Fruits — cantaloupe, grapes, and berries.
- ◆ Carbohydrates — rice, corn chips, potato chips, pop-
corn, and graham crackers.
- ◆ All nuts.
- ◆ Miscellaneous — eggs, nonmilk chocolate, and Jell-O.

Water was found to produce the least gas of all. The following foods were moderately flatugenic for Mr. Sutalf: pastries, potatoes, eggplant, citrus fruit, apples, and bread. And these foods — in Mr. Sutalf's case, at least — were extremely flatugenic: milk and milk products, onions, beans, celery, carrots, raisins, bananas, apricots, prune juice, pretzels, bagels, wheat germ, and brussels sprouts.

Further testing, the article noted, will be necessary to determine whether this diet, which worked for one patient, will benefit other flatulent individuals.

In 1981, a study by Isabel H. Anderson, Allen S. Levine, and Dr. Levitt suggested that flatulence may be caused by the small bowel's inability to absorb and digest the gluten in ordinary wheat flour. This form of starch may then pass into the intestinal tract where it feeds gas-producing bacteria. Eighteen healthy volunteers ate meals of white bread, macaroni, bread made from brown-rice flour, bread made from low-gluten wheat flour, and bread made from low-gluten wheat flour with gluten added.

The investigators then measured the amount of hydrogen produced in the breath of the volunteers. An increase in breath hydrogen after eating carbohydrates indicated that absorption in the small bowel was incomplete. The study showed that breath hydrogen increased substantially after the subjects ate bread made from white, all-purpose wheat flour. Bread made from the other kinds of flours caused little or no increase in breath hydrogen. The finding that gluten may be a culprit in producing flatulence is consistent with the Levitt-Sutalf study, which found that a low-wheat diet reduced flatulence. Despite such discoveries, it has still not been established to science's satisfaction whether diet, swallowed air, or other factors are the major source of intestinal gas.

During times of stress, excitement, tension, anxiety, or aggravation, many people gulp air. The turbulence in their guts reflects emotional, not organic disturbance. Many people feel the churning when they are worried, angry, or faced with situations and people they don't like. This type of attack is often accompanied by shortness of breath, pounding of the heart, and chest pains — symptoms frighteningly like a heart attack. People who suffer frequent "gas attacks" also tend to be chronically tired. Stress also causes hypermotility, a condition in which food and gases no longer pass through the intestine in an orderly fashion, causing spasms or cramps frequently mislabeled as "gas pains." Still, these pains from gut distension can be relieved by reducing the volume of intestinal gas, even though excessive gas is not the primary problem.

High altitude also poses some problems for the flatulent: the volume of intestinal gas doubles at fifteen thousand feet, and increases nearly eightfold at forty thousand feet, making flatus among the more noxious side effects experienced by the astronauts. The increase is similar to balloon expansion at high altitudes. Gases trapped in the gut expand in inverse proportion to the atmospheric pressure outside the body. Pilots have long experienced pain caused by flatulence at high altitudes. Among the factors that make it worse are eating gas-forming foods such as carbohydrates and milk, irritating foods like cabbage and spices, and foods to which you may be allergic.

To cut down on gas production:

♦ Eat foods that are easily digested, especially those that are bland or low in fat.
♦ Avoid foods that contain gas, or may cause it to form, such as onions, beans, garlic, cabbage, carbohydrates, milk, milkshakes, meringues, soufflés, and carbonated beverages.
♦ Exercise daily: walk whenever possible, climb stairs, jog, and avoid sitting for hours at a time.
♦ On long car trips, stop and take a walk every hour.
♦ If you are an air swallower, correct the factors that make it worse: ill-fitting dentures, nasal congestion, smoking, chewing gum, gasping, talking and eating too fast, and sipping through straws.
♦ Try to eat more slowly. Fletcherize.
♦ Stop eating when you feel uncomfortable.
♦ If you are nervous, try to discover why, and avoid stressful situations.

If you already have gas pains, relieve them by rocking back and forth with your knees held close to your chest, and let the gas pass into the mattress. Try lying prone over some pillows, or — if you are athletic — standing on your head. This works because gas tends to rise. The less athletic can try a modified headstand: bend over the edge of a bed or padded table with your legs on the flat surface and hands on the floor. In this position, your body, face downward, forms a right angle. A heating pad applied to the abdomen may also provide some relief.

These measures generally work better than many widely advertised, over-the-counter medications for stomach and gas upsets. Gas sufferers often dose themselves with antacids, which do not help. Bicarbonate of soda helps the intestine expel gas, but should be used only in emergencies because it can contribute to high blood pressure and disturb body metabolism. However, the drug simethicone may bring some relief. It is a derivative of silicone, which is used in industry to disperse foam. Simethicone does the same thing in the digestive tract by breaking open gas bubbles and moving them along. A few over-the-counter liquid antacid preparations — Di-Gel, for example — contain simethicone. Activated charcoal tablets have long been used to absorb intestinal gas, but a Food and Drug Administration panel of experts recently reported that their continued use could deplete certain essential nutrients, and counteract the effects of other drugs you might be taking. Nor has activated charcoal been proven effective against intestinal gas. The panel members therefore recommend that activated charcoal be taken no longer than seven days, and that the dosage be limited to ten grams daily, unless your doctor advises differently.

For centuries, authors and scholars have pondered how to deal with flatulence. Robert Burton, an Elizabethan scholar, recommended in *Anatomy of Melancholy* that hypochondriacs tormented by wind should attach a pair of bellows to a clyster pipe, insert it in the "fundament," and draw forth the wind. In his "Letter to the Royal Academy of Brussels," Benjamin Franklin wrote:

It is universally well known, that in digesting our common Food, there is created or produced in the Bowels of human creatures, a great quantity of Wind. . . . Were it not for the odiously offensive Smell accompanying such escapes, polite People would probably be under no more Restraint in discharging such Wind in Company, than they are in spitting or in blowing their Noses. . . . A few stems of Asparagus eaten, shall give our Urine a disagreeable Odour; and a Pill of Turpentine no bigger than a Pea, shall bestow on it the pleasing Smell of Violets. And why should it be thought more impossible in Nature, to find Means of making a Perfume of our *Wind* than of our *Water?*

Other great men of letters have dealt with the subject no less imaginatively. In *1601*, Mark Twain described a "Conversation as it was at the Social Fireside in the time of the Tudors":

Yesternight took her Majestie, ye Queene, a fantasie such as she sometimes hath, and hadde to her closet certeain that do write playes, books & such like. . . . In ye heate of ye talke, it befel that one did breake wynde, yielding an exceeding mightie and distressful stinke, whereat all did laffe full sore, and then:

YE QUEENE: Verily, in mine eight and sixty yeares have I not heard the fellow to this fartte. . . . Prithee, let ye author confess ye offspring. (Whereupon each member of the company denied authorship until, at last, Sir Walter Raleigh owned up.)

In modern times, J.P. Donleavy advises in *The Unexpurgated Code*, "Never admit to farting even if there are only two of you." Or say, "My soul speaks when my mouth knows the moment is too divine for words." Donleavy further advises that "Farting is fine while shooting but not while stalking."

One reason that flatulence is a problem is that society pressures us to suppress the natural act. According to psychoanalytic theory, this rule was authored by parents who allow themselves the privilege of passing gas, but strictly deny it to their children. Such social conventions often cause people to try to suppress gas and to disguise it, for example, by simultaneously sneezing. This does little to conceal gas that smells, so a true course of prevention must shun foods that lend farts their distinctive odor. In general, carbohydrates produce the least aromatic gas and, as Benjamin Franklin noted in his letter to the Royal Academy:

> He that dines on stale Flesh, especially with much Addition of Onions, shall be able to afford a Stink that no Company can tolerate; while he that has liv'd for some time on Vegetables only, shall have that Breath so pure as to be insensible to the most delicate Noses . . ."

Eructation, Etc.

When your car backfires, it usually means the electrical timing is off. When *you* backfire, whether through the carburetor or the muffler, it may mean that you have swallowed air. Air can pass from mouth to anus in thirty to forty-five minutes, or from stomach to mouth even faster. Whichever way it goes, let it.

In 1973, the *British Medical Journal* described what could happen if you suppress this natural force. A man leaned across the table as his bridge partner lit his cigarette. Suddenly he felt a belch coming on, but suppressed it:

> Unfortunately, he attempted to do this discreetly through his nose. He astonished the company by producing two fan-shaped flames from his nostrils. His partner, who accompanied him to the casualty department, described the incident as 'just like a dragon, doctor.'

In another incident, a man described as "prone to violent and foul-smelling eructations," cupped his hands to light a cigarette in a movie theater and belched. To the astonishment of those seated around him, there was a flash and a sharp explosion. The cigarette shot out of his mouth and landed several rows of seats over. In a similar case, a man's breath caught fire one night when he was blowing out a match. Another man belched while blowing out a match, which he had struck in order to read his watch. His breath caught fire and his moustache was burned.

As noted earlier, intestinal gas contains varying proportions of oxygen, nitrogen, carbon dioxide, hydrogen, and methane. This makes it so flammable, regardless of which end emits it, that it has caused explosions when it has come into contact with anesthetics during surgical procedures.

Belching has other features as well. It is good for relieving gas pains in babies, in which case it is called "burping." And it is also good for boat bottoms, if *Boating* magazine can be believed. In a recent promotion letter, the magazine recommended adding ground red pepper to cheap copper bottom paint on the theory that it will *burp* the barnacles to death. "Don't laugh," the letter said, "One boat owner who tried it reported fourteen months in South Florida waters without a barnacle."

In humans, belching is caused by swallowing air with food, drinks (especially the carbonated variety), and saliva, or by gulping air down alone. In nervous people, belching is called *eructatio nervosa*. Belching may occur when the stomach empties slowly because of a blockage in the pyloric valve. This traps food in the stomach long enough to ferment and form gases.

For other people, the problem is not belching, but the inability to belch. Their esophageal sphincter is so tight that gas cannot pass upward. Swallowed air may then collect in the stomach and form an air bubble which sometimes causes heartburn. The more air you swallow, the bigger the bubble becomes and the more bloated you feel. The only way out is through the tailpipe.

Belching usually occurs involuntarily after meals as you release some of the air swallowed with food. However, certain people can belch at will. This relieves the pressure, but not the symptom itself. To prevent burps and belches, it is necessary to eat and chew more slowly, and to discover whether anxiety may be adding to the problem. In other words, slow down, calm down, and do not squelch a belch. Orientals consider belching after a meal complimentary to your host, and do not disfavor belching in public. If anybody objects, just tell them:

It's better to belch,
And bear the shame,
Than squelch a belch,
And bear the pain!

Gurgles and Growls

Borborygmus (musical stomach) is the sound of air and liquid from digesting food sloshing around inside your stomach and intestine. For most people, a rumbling gut is a normal occurrence. You may think it is caused by "hunger pangs." Strictly speaking, however, a noisy gut is not caused by hunger, although the anticipation of eating can generate peristalsis and subsequent borborygmic rumblings.

One fourteen-year-old girl had borborygmus so badly that it threatened her budding career as a concert pianist. When she sought medical help, X rays revealed no tumor, ulcer, or obstruction. Under the fluoroscope, doctors could see that sudden, sharp contractions were forcing fluids noisily upward. This revealed the mechanics, but not the origin, of her intestinal rumbles. Doctors finally discovered that they were caused by nervous swallowing of air. A tranquilizer soothed her gut and saved her career. Other causes of borborygmus include ulcers, tumors, dysentery, structural abnormalities, gastrointestinal bleeding, and inability to digest milk and milk products.

If you want to tone down your tummy, lie on your back or your right side, apply pressure to your abdomen, and avoid carbonated beverages. Eating may also help to relieve borborygmus.

In most cases, the sounds and sloshings of borborygmus are perfectly normal. High-pitched sounds mean air or fluid is moving under high pressure through a narrow passage such as the small intestine. Lower rumbles mean air and fluid are being pushed through a large passage under low pressure. So the next time you hear a stomach growl — whether it's yours or somebody else's — don't be embarrassed. Relax and enjoy the stomach's concert, for it has a music all its own.

Hiccups

Hiccups are really a respiratory problem. However, indigestion and other gut reactions can cause these spasms of the diaphragm, a domed wall of muscle and tendons just above the stomach that separates the chest from the abdominal cavity. The windpipe snaps shut, suddenly stops the intake of breath, and causes the gasping sound of the hiccup. Hiccup spasms may occur as often as forty to one hundred times per minute.

Although the basic cause of the hiccup remains a medical mystery, indigestion can trigger the ordinary case of hiccups, which lasts five or ten minutes. Other causes include excessive eating, drinking, smoking, swallowing air, or gulping hot or cold liquids. Disease in any part of the body — stroke, heart attack, pneumonia, hernia, diabetes, influenza, bronchitis, brain tumor, or skull fracture — can cause hiccups, as can sudden fright or severe mental shock. One man who had been married and childless for two years developed hiccups after receiving a medical report confirming that his semen was sterile. An arcane bit of medical information — known to medical students as "a pearl" passed along by one of their professors — is that a hair in your ear, just touching against the tympanic membrane inside, can cause hiccups. In such cases, the cure is to remove the hair. But not all hiccups are silenced so simply.

The 1981 edition of the *Guinness Book of World Records* reports that "the longest recorded attack of hiccoughs was that afflicting Charles Osborne (born 1894) of Anthon, Iowa, from 1922 to date. He contracted it when slaughtering a hog." *Guinness* also reports that a young man was admitted to the infirmary at Newcastle upon Tyne in England on March 25, 1769, because he was suffering from hiccoughs which could be heard at a range of more than a mile. Many patients whose hiccups (or hiccoughs) have lasted days or weeks have been admitted to hospitals in imminent danger of death from lack of oxygen, heart failure, or extreme debilitation. These are extraordinary cases. For most people, an attack of hiccups is over in less than an hour.

Hiccup remedies include holding your breath, drinking water, breathing into a paper bag, or having someone frighten you, with variations such as drinking water by sipping from the far side of the glass or swallowing with a pencil between your teeth. Other remedies include tickling your nose until you sneeze, pulling out your tongue, or making yourself vomit. These measures work because they interrupt the reflex that perpetuates the hiccups. A recently rediscovered cure for hiccups is a teaspoonful of white granulated sugar, swallowed dry.

When hiccups last longer than a few hours or recur with frequency, you should see a doctor since a more elaborate treatment may be necessary. These include muscle relaxants, central nervous system stimulants, tranquilizers, antiepileptic drugs, whiffs of ether, and even hypnosis. In extreme cases of hiccups, your doctor may inject special drugs into your neck to block the phrenic nerves which control the diaphragm where hiccup spasms occur. As a last resort, one of the phrenic nerves may have to be severed surgically.

Hiccups are a peculiar phenomenon. Unlike the cough, sneeze, and belch — which, in turn, clear your throat, open your nose, and ease your bloated stomach — the hiccup does you no good at all.

Halitosis

As a 1873 dental journal noted, ". . . no one detects the smell he is used to, and by consequence, since each one is accustomed to his own breath, he will regard it as odorless, though its vapors be loaded with a dozen different stenches." (Dentists, the journal added, are among the worst offenders.)

Halitosis (bad breath) or fetor oris (*very* bad breath), may originate in your mouth, lungs, breathing passages, or nose. But eighty-five to ninety percent of it originates in your mouth, where it is caused by decaying food, stagnating saliva, dental caries, bleeding gums, periodontal disease, and plaque (invisible bacterial accumulations on the teeth).

In addition, a coated tongue can cause bad breath, especially the back portion, which emits the strongest odor. Dry mouth and breathing from your mouth also cause foul breath because the saliva dries and cannot wash your teeth and mouth free of bacteria and their smelly by-products.

Bad breath in the morning, sometimes called "bird cage breath," may mean a sinus or adenoid infection, or tonsillitis. However, you may have bad breath in the morning simply because your tongue has been inactive all night, and saliva has not done its job of keeping your oral cavity clean.

Halitosis is also caused by dirty dentures, laxatives, smoking, drinking alcohol, canker sores, postnasal drip, throat infections, bronchitis, lung abscess, or malignant tumors. Bad breath may occur when you are under psychological stress, or when you are hungry. The longer the interval between meals, the worse the problem becomes. When food passes over your tongue, it cleans off putrefied surface film and stimulates the flow of saliva. So if you skip breakfast, you may have bad breath even though you brushed your teeth.

About fifteen percent of breath odor originates in the body. If you eat high-fat foods (especially milk and butter fats), refined sugar, and white flour, you are more prone to halitosis. During digestion, certain chemicals produced by these foods are picked up in the blood and eliminated through the lungs and mouth. For example, if capsules containing onion or garlic are swallowed without chewing, the odor will soon be detected on your breath and may last for seventy-two hours. That is why mouthwash won't help such cases. As Shakespeare advises in *A Midsummer Night's Dream* (Act 4, scene 2, line 40): "Eat no onions nor garlic, for we are to utter sweet breath."

Most cases of halitosis can be cured if you:

♦ Brush your teeth, gums, and tongue as far back as possible three times a day. (The Romans used iron tongue scrapers; all you need is a soft-bristle toothbrush.)
♦ Suck sugarless lozenges to help increase the flow of saliva between brushings.
♦ Visit your dentist regularly to have decay-causing plaque removed, and control it between visits by brushing and flossing between the teeth.
♦ Do not use mouthwashes. These products do little more than mask halitosis for a few hours.
♦ A final remedy for halitosis is eating.
♦ Remember, many cases of halitosis go untreated, but they seldom go unnoticed.

PART III

Battle of the Bowel

CHAPTER 9

North of the Navel

IN THE EIGHTEENTH century, James Boswell wrote that ". . . he who does not mind his belly will hardly mind anything else." The twentieth-century American has a different approach:

AUTHOR: Do you listen to your stomach?
FRIEND: Sure!
AUTHOR: Then what do you do?
FRIEND: I tell it to shut up!

Small wonder that stomach troubles plague so many people. According to the British epidemiologists Drs. Denis P. Burkitt and Neil S. Painter, a disturbing number of digestive problems have made a debut in this country during the last half century. Diverticular disease has been a major health problem only in the last sixty years, and hiatus hernia has been recognized as a common condition only during the last thirty.

Moreover, hiatus hernia, gallstones, appendicitis, diverticular disease, hemorrhoids, and cancer of the colon and rectum — so prevalent in industrialized nations — are virtually unknown in developing countries. But when these countries begin to adopt the diets and lifestyles of Western civilization, the prevalence of these conditions increases. Why?

Drs. Burkitt and Painter believe — and the evidence supporting them is growing stronger — that many digestive diseases that afflict so-called "civilized" countries stem from the kinds of foods you eat, especially the low-fiber diets that prevail in the United States. Other theories hold that you are more susceptible to these diseases because of diet and the way you deal with stress. These are the factors that have such a large influence when your gullet won't function properly, or digestive juices burn holes in your stomach, or your liver's chemical factory shuts down, or gallstones form. Several problems can afflict your upper gastrointestinal tract — the part that lies north of the navel — including hiatus hernia, ulcers, cirrhosis of the liver, hepatitis, gallbladder disease, and pancreatitis.

Hiatus Hernia

Also known as hiatal hernia, this is one of the diseases that is virtually unknown in countries where diets are high in cereal and other fiber. Dietary fiber eases the passage of bowel movements. Straining at stool, on the other hand, causes increased abdominal pressures that could, according to Dr. Burkitt's theory of "pressure diseases," lead to hiatal hernia.

To understand why this is so, consider your anatomy. After food and water enter your stomach, a special valve at the bottom of your esophagus — known as the lower esophageal sphincter (LES) — shuts. This valve keeps food and stomach secretions from backing up into your esophagus and mouth.

The esophageal valve is located in an opening through your diaphragm, which separates your chest cavity (and esophagus) from your abdominal cavity (and stomach). Where the esophagus and stomach join, there is a teardrop-shaped opening in the diaphragm called the hiatus.

Sometimes when your hiatus is too large, your stomach can slide up, then down into your chest cavity. This condition is called hiatus hernia, *hernia* referring to the protrusion of an organ — in this case, the stomach — from the cavity where it is normally located. In seventy-five to ninety-five percent of all hiatus hernias, part of the stomach slides straight up through the opening into the chest. In a small number called "rolling" hiatus hernias, the stomach slides up through the hiatus and flops forward into the chest cavity.

The protruding portion of the stomach is under far more pressure than the rest of your stomach, just as the part of a balloon you squeeze between your fingers is under greater pressure than the rest of the balloon. Despite this pressure, hiatus hernia usually causes no problem as long as your esophageal valve works. This explains why most people who have a hiatus hernia do not even know it. But when pressures from the stomach are stronger than the esophageal valve, the valve may allow digestive juices to back up from your stomach into your esophagus, where they will attack the sensitive mucous membrane lining its walls. This backflow, or reflux, as it is called, may cause severe heartburn, described in Chapter 5 as the burning pain, pressure, and sour regurgitation that usually strikes within a half hour after a meal. Or the lining of your esophagus may become inflamed, leading to a more serious condition known as reflux esophagitis.

While hiatus hernia itself is painless, esophagitis can cause pains so sharp that some people confuse them with angina pectoris, a form of heart disease marked by severe chest pain. Until recently, many people with hiatus hernia needlessly became "cardiac cripples" because their disorder mimicked heart disease. One eighty-year-old woman, even though she knew the severe pains that woke her up one night were probably caused by her hiatus hernia, could scarcely contain her fears. She telephoned her doctor, who spent forty-five minutes reassuring her that she was not having a heart attack, and that her fears stemmed more from being alone than from being in pain.

Problems that accompany hiatus hernia can be triggered by coughing, vomiting, straining at stool, sudden physical exertion, pregnancy, obesity, or the collection of fluid in the abdomen. These all exert pressure on the stomach and abdomen. The "heartburn habits" mentioned in Chapter 5 can aggravate these problems. So can emotional stress since tension increases the secretion of gastric juices.

Can hiatus hernia be prevented? Probably not, since it apparently occurs when muscles in your diaphragm slacken with age. About half of the people over age forty in this country are thought to have hiatus hernia, especially if they are overweight or have borne a child. And everyone who lives long enough will probably develop at least a small hiatus hernia. But most of these people will never develop heartburn. Only when hiatus hernia is complicated by heartburn and esophagitis is treatment necessary. In fact, neglect of these conditions could lead to scarring and narrowing of the esophagus, and possibly even to an inability to swallow solid food.

These complications need not occur if you give heartburn and esophagitis "careful handling" at the outset:

- Take antacids as prescribed by your doctor to neutralize stomach acid and reduce inflammation of the esophagus.
- Avoid foods and other substances that are known to weaken the esophageal valve. These include tobacco, alcohol, coffee, tea, chocolate, garlic, onion, highly spiced and fatty foods, and peppermint.
- Lose weight if you are too heavy.
- Sleep with the head of your bed raised four to ten inches.
- Eat smaller meals more frequently, and don't eat so much that you feel stuffed.
- Don't smoke, especially if you have "smoker's cough."
- Don't go to bed on a full stomach.
- Don't exercise immediately after eating.
- Don't wear tight clothing.
- Don't bend forward to scrub floors or weed the garden.

About ninety percent of the cases of heartburn and other problems caused by hiatus hernia respond to these commonsense measures. But if your case doesn't respond, your doctor may prescribe atropine, belladonna, or other drugs that block acid secretion in the stomach. Several new drugs, including cimetidine, are being prescribed by physicians for esophagitis even though the Food and Drug Administration (FDA) has not yet approved them for this use. There is nothing wrong with the practice; it merely means the FDA has neither *approved* nor *disapproved* this particular use for these drugs. Cimetidine has been widely used in Europe, but because the FDA is often slow to accept evidence from any but United States researchers, there has been a "drug lag" in this country.

As a last resort, your physician may recommend surgery to correct hiatus hernia. Surgery is necessary if there is any danger that gastric juices might enter and damage your lungs, or if the herniated stomach's blood supply is cut off and the tissue begins to die. In recent years, several new operations have been devised to return the displaced stomach to its normal position and provide a flap valve to replace the esophageal valve or reinforce its action.

Other disorders of the esophagus include dysphagia, or difficulty with swallowing. You may take swallowing so much for granted that it is hard to imagine anybody having trouble with it. But dysphagia is more common than many people realize. It is usually caused by the combination of esophagitis and achalasia — a failure of the muscles of the esophageal sphincter to relax after something has been swallowed — which creates an intensely uncomfortable feeling of "something sticking." Dysphagia may be caused by cancer or by tumors that squeeze the esophagus shut from the outside. Sometimes a constricting "ring," or narrow place in the esophagus, interferes with swallowing. Your doctor may prescribe "bougienage," or dilatation of the esophagus, to open the passageway. You may not like it, but the alternative is surgery.

Emotional upsets can also cause difficulty swallowing. Dr. Stewart Wolf, who followed the case of Tom, conducted tests in the early 1950s of the swallowing patterns of patients under stress. Initially, one woman could swallow liquid barium in less than thirty seconds. But when Dr. Wolf mentioned her spouse, with whom she was having marital difficulties, the barium took fifteen minutes to go down. It is hard to swallow when you feel grief, because crying causes your throat membranes to swell and become tender, so that you cannot even breathe normally. Often when you have just suffered a severe emotional shock, well-meaning friends insist that you "eat something to keep up your strength." But you are apt to find that food "sticks" at the back of your mouth and even makes you choke. You are better off fasting until you regain your swallowing mechanism.

The muscles of your esophagus are very susceptible to the power of suggestion. Sometimes the fear that "this pill just won't go down" can be self-fulfilling. There are other problems with "popping" pills. Some researchers at Temple University who investigated some of the causes of inflammation of the esophagus, tested how long it takes various liquids, tablets, or capsules to clear the esophagus when sitting or lying down. They found that most gelatin capsules went down in fifteen seconds if taken with a water chaser. But a capsule taken with no water at all took up to one hour to clear the esophagus in more than half the subjects. Yet ninety percent of them were unaware that the capsule had gone down only part way and might be dissolving in the wrong section of their digestive tracts. When you take a pill, sit up and take it with several swallows of liquid as a chaser. Don't take pills with sodas or acid fruit juices. They may make the drug dissolve too quickly in your stomach rather than in your intestines, where most drugs can be absorbed more easily.

Ulcers

Mary Queen of Scots — as if she didn't have enough problems with her cousin Queen Elizabeth, assorted husbands, political crises, and eventual mental collapse — also suffered from a peptic ulcer. For at least twenty-five years of her life, she endured abdominal pain, attacks of vomiting, and several times almost died from profuse bleeding. There was no surgery for ulcers in those days, and it says much for her courage and constitution that she recovered from repeated attacks. In the last four years before her execution, her ulcer apparently remained healed.

Napoleon also suffered from a peptic ulcer that leaked

blood for years and caused a lifetime of poor health. Napoleon's ulcer, unlike Mary's, not only bled, but eventually perforated. It ate a hole clear through his stomach, spilling blood and acids, and causing infection throughout his abdominal cavity. He died in exile on the island of St. Helena, of what he described as "a sharp, piercing pain that cut into me like a razor." Though Napoleon's doctor was convinced that his patient's trouble was of neurotic origin, the Emperor was actually dying of perforated peptic ulcer, hemorrhage, and peritonitis. The autopsy report described "an ulcer which penetrated the coats of the stomach . . . one inch from the pylorus, sufficient to allow passage of the little finger. . . . The stomach was found nearly filled with a large quantity of fluid resembling coffee grounds."

Ulcer patients once faced a lifetime of pain, bland diets, and the possibility that their ulcers would ultimately perforate. No longer. Today, people realize that ulcers are no longer a disaster, thanks to some amazing medical advances in treatment and detection, plus the fact that ulcers tend to heal spontaneously. Ulcers resemble large canker sores. They are eroded areas that have been eaten away (autodigested) by powerful digestive acids, which, in the healthy stomach, slip harmlessly over a protective coating of mucus. Although ulcers are usually smaller than a dime, some are the diameter of a Ping-Pong or even a tennis ball. They can occur one at a time, or in clusters by the dozens.

Ulcers that occur in the lining of your stomach — usually in the end portion near the pyloric valve that leads to the duodenum — are called gastric ulcers. The vast majority of ulcers, however, occur in the first part of your small intestine. This area, the duodenum, lacks the stomach's protective mucus "undercoating," and can erode under the outflow of digestive juices from the stomach. Duodenal ulcers are common among people in their twenties and thirties, while gastric ulcers are more likely to strike those over age forty.

If ulcers are ignored, eventually one cell too many is eaten away and perforation may occur. Stomach contents seep, then spill through the punched-out hole, spreading infection throughout your abdominal cavity. But today peritonitis can be controlled with antibiotics.

Ulcers are an ancient ailment. St. Paul, who complained of recurrent pain "like a thorn in the flesh," probably had an ulcer. Pliny, the Roman author and statesman, reportedly used crushed coral to relieve his abdominal pain, and Paracelsus, the medieval physician who was also known as Theophrastus Bombastus von Hohenheim, used crushed pearls.

In 350 B.C., a medical writer described the symptoms of ulcers: a steady, gnawing pain at the tip of the breastbone that strikes thirty minutes to two hours after a meal, and is usually relieved by eating. Nocturnal pain between midnight and 2:00 A.M. is common because an empty stomach is more vulnerable to burning digestive acids. The pain may take the form of a warm or gnawing feeling akin to a hunger pang in the stomach, or of a "gas pocket," or of vague discomfort anywhere in the abdomen.

Sometimes ulcer pain is confused with heartburn. Ulcer pain is usually more severe and lasts longer, frequently occurring day after day. It tends to strike at the same hour — just *before* a meal — while heartburn and indigestion occur *after* meals. It is important to recognize symptoms before an ulcer begins to bleed or bore a hole in your stomach. The problem is that some ulcers cause no pain at all, and are impossible to detect until extensive damage is done. As a general rule, bleeding ulcers do not cause pain (possibly because of the buffering effect of blood), and painful ulcers do not bleed. In either case, the average patient may suffer from an ulcer for two years before it is diagnosed accurately.

The first sign of serious trouble may be bleeding from the intestinal tract as the eroded area cuts through a blood vessel. This might cause you to suddenly vomit material that resembles coffee grounds, or to pass bloody or dark, tarry stools. If this happens, you will hardly need to be told: see a doctor.

Doctors know how ulcers behave, who is at risk, and some spectacular ways to treat and prevent them, but nobody knows what causes ulcers. It *is* known that stomach acid is necessary for ulcers to occur. "No acid, no ulcer," the saying goes. According to one theory, people who develop ulcers tend to secrete more than a normal amount of hydrochloric acid and pepsin, the enzyme that helps break up food and prepare it for digestion. But it is also possible that people who develop ulcers are abnormally sensitive even to normal amounts of these corrosive gastric juices.

Ulcers are considered a disease of modern civilization. Duodenal ulcers, the more common of the two types, were virtually unknown in Europe prior to 1900, and only seventy cases were reported in England during the entire nineteenth century. Around World War I, duodenal ulcers started increasing and, by the beginning of World War II, were very common. More recently, ulcers have become prevalent in Japan, while they have declined overall in the United States. Although about twenty million Americans — or about ten percent of the population — have had, or currently have, an ulcer, the incidence in the United States has dropped to less than one in twenty men, while rates for women have correspondingly increased. Scotland's rate is higher than England's, suggesting that peptic ulcers may decline once people have adapted to the stresses of industrialization. In the nineteenth century, men developed five to ten times as many duodenal ulcers as women. Today, the sex ratio among duodenal ulcer victims is less than two to one. Women develop as many gastric ulcers as men, and both gastric and duodenal ulcers are rising among the elderly of both sexes.

It has recently been discovered that ulcers tend to run in families, and are about three times more common in close relatives of a person with ulcers than in the general population. The portrait of the typical ulcer victim is also changing. Classically, people with ulcers were labeled as ambitious, high-pressure businessmen with tight schedules and uptight personalities. Not so, recent studies say. High-stress jobs are no more likely to produce ulcers than boring, production-line occupations. Garbage collectors, farmers, and factory workers are as vulnerable as corporate presidents.

The idea that emotional upsets cause ulcers was first suggested by Amatus Lusitanus, a sixteenth-century Spanish physician whose old friend and fellow physician, Azariah dei Rossi, was being persecuted by Spanish Inquisitors for being a Jew. Amatus blamed his friend's stomach distresses on the tensions and terrors of living under the Inquisition, and told

Azariah to sleep more and study less. Amatus also prescribed a special diet of cooked fruit, vegetables, and chicken soup. Azariah survived not only his ulcer but the Inquisition as well, and enjoyed good health for another thirty years.

When a stressful situation continues long enough, your ability to adapt to it declines (as explained in Chapter 3), along with your ability to resist diseases such as ulcers. A complex series of physiological events can cause an increase in the secretion of gastric juices in your stomach. After days and weeks, the overproduction of highly acidic gastric juice may activate, reactivate, or cause an ulcer to bleed. This alarm reaction may be triggered by temperature changes, muscular exertion and fatigue, or by anxiety, hostility, and rage.

The link between hostility and overproduction of gastric juices applies even to animals hunting in the wild. They must pursue, fight, kill, and eat in rapid sequence. To do all of this quickly, the animal's stomach steps up its gastric secretions and muscular contractions when it receives the signal that the hunt — or battle — is on.

In one classic study, personality tests designed to predict which Army inductees would develop ulcers during basic training identified a so-called "ulcer personality." It was defined as a person who strongly needs the approval of others, who develops deep resentments, and who has great difficulty expressing those resentments in a socially acceptable manner.

Another study described duodenal ulcer patients as people who are overly diligent, unable to say "no," and who need to be loved in order to feel secure. They try to gain this by being clean, tidy, and hard-working. When they fail to achieve love no matter what they do, they express their unrequited needs through their stomachs. In the psychiatric view, this leads to a constant state of hyperactivity and acid secretion in that organ, as if in expectation of food. The stomach behaves as it does during digestion, when, in fact, there is no food for stomach secretions to digest. Thus, a "nervous" stomach that produces too much gastric juice can trigger heartburn, esophagitis, and, eventually, a painful and incapacitating ulcer.

Some people question whether conflicts over wanting to be loved could stimulate stomach secretions and all the consequent effects. There is, however, ample evidence that upset, anxious people — whether their anxiety stems from feeling unloved or from other personal problems — secrete more digestive juice not only at mealtime, but throughout the day. Studies have shown, for example, that gastric acid levels of students are significantly higher during exam periods than at other times. Other studies, as mentioned in Chapter 3, show that tissue damage from ulcers tends to become worse during the early stages of psychotherapy when bottled-up emotions are brought to the level of consciousness. Once you are aware of these feelings, the theory goes, the physical symptoms of ulcers and other such diseases improve as treatment is directed at the emotional roots of the illness.

In his textbook *Clinical Gastroenterology* (N.Y.: Macmillan, 1977), Dr. Howard M. Spiro describes what happened when one patient, a forty-year-old physician, repressed his emotions. "For many years," Dr. Spiro writes, "he had been a curmudgeon, chasing some patients from his office, giving salty advice to others, and generally raising cain." Then, one day, the physician decided that life was short and he would be kind to everybody, no matter how he felt. As Dr. Spiro tells it:

> Exactly on the day that he made that decision, he first suffered severe ulcer pain. . . . He finally came to the hospital with intractable pain from a posterior penetrating duodenal ulcer for a decision as to whether he needed a gastric resection. Faced with the possibility of losing his stomach, the patient recognized exactly what had happened and what his cure should be.

He went back to his curmudgeonly ways, and soon afterward, his ulcer stopped causing him pain and did not recur. "Unfortunately," Dr. Spiro concludes, "not everyone can give vent to his feelings as easily as the successful physician."

Experience shows that only duodenal, not gastric, ulcers, may be caused by emotional factors. Yet even in cases of duodenal ulcer, there is still no hard proof that stress is a primary cause. Many of the emotional roots of ulcers remain to be discovered. As Dr. Harold P. Roth, authority on digestive diseases from the National Institutes of Health, states, "Maybe we just haven't studied it in the right way." Whatever the cause, an important, but often difficult, part of the treatment of an ulcer is the reduction of worry and tension.

Other factors besides stress appear to be associated with ulcers. So-called acute ulcers can occur in association with abdominal surgery, shock and head injury, or some other acute disease or illness. Curling's ulcer, for example, occurs about seventy-two hours after a massive burn, and Cushing's ulcer frequently accompanies central nervous system disease. Steroid ulcer, another type of acute ulcer, often occurs in persons who take steroids for rheumatoid arthritis.

Smoking increases the risk of developing ulcers because it inhibits the pancreas from secreting chemicals that neutralize stomach acids entering the duodenum. This finding provides an explanation for the increase in ulcers among women: more of them smoke. Smokers of both sexes suffer twice the rate of duodenal ulcers as nonsmokers, and develop gastric ulcers three to four times as often.

Regular use of aspirin is also known to triple the risk of developing gastric ulcers. Ulcers occurred six times more often among twenty-five hundred recovered heart-attack victims who took aspirin as a treatment for hardening of the arteries than among an equal number of heart patients who took pills that lacked aspirin's active ingredients. Animal studies show that when regular doses of aspirin and alcohol are combined, they produce bleeding ulcers. If taken separately, the same doses would not produce any damage. Claims are being made for a new "gentler" aspirin that ulcer patients may be able to tolerate. Recent studies show that enteric-coated aspirin, designed to dissolve in the small intestine instead of the stomach, appears to provide some insulation from the harmful effects of aspirin. Buffered aspirin tablets offer little or no protection to the stomach lining.

One theory suggests that because alcohol and coffee increase the amount of gastric juices in the stomach, those who consume them in large quantities are more likely to get ulcers. Other studies do not confirm this finding. If you have an ulcer, there is little question that, until it heals, you should avoid these substances, especially on an empty stomach.

Diet is still an important part of ulcer treatment, although the traditional "baby food" diet is now considered passé. Researchers have discovered that bland foods like cream of wheat for breakfast, cream soup for lunch, and poached flounder for dinner do nothing to help heal an ulcer, although they may, for some people, relieve symptoms — no small benefit for people with ulcer pain. Milk, once thought to relieve ulcers by neutralizing stomach juices, apparently is more soothing to the mind than the body. Recent studies show that although it relieves ulcer pain for ten to fifteen minutes, its *net* effect is to *increase* stomach acidity.

In general, if you have an ulcer, you should eat frequently during the day. What you eat is strictly a personal matter, determined by you, your stomach, and your doctor. If foods you are accustomed to don't bother you, by all means, eat them. But if your ulcer is acting up, you might feel better switching to poached flounder and other bland foods for awhile. If you would like a helping hand, the American Digestive Disease Society publishes a series of dietary plans, one of which, the "ulcer" diet, can help you find your own food patterns and discover which foods are good for — as well as *to* — your ulcer (see Appendix A).

Antacids remain a classic treatment for ulcers because they neutralize stomach secretions. Of the more than five hundred different antacids on the market, some types are safer and more effective than others. For example, antacids like Maalox and Gelusil are not absorbed through the walls of the stomach, and do not stimulate the stomach to secrete acid. Liquid antacids work better than tablets, which must be chewed thoroughly to a fine powder to effectively coat your stomach lining. Take antacids one to three hours after meals, at bedtime, and any other time you feel ulcer pain.

Here are some other ways to take care of your ulcer until it heals:

♦ Avoid anything that damages your stomach or makes it produce more acid: cigarettes, aspirin, hard liquor, coffee, tea, hot and spicy foods, and carbonated drinks with caffeine.

◆ Learn to handle stress and anger. If pressures are too great, learn to blow off steam rather than store it up, or back off and give yourself a chance to say, "Whew!"

◆ Don't start the day with a cigarette and coffee for breakfast, especially not the day you're scheduled for a stressful meeting with your boss.

◆ Don't take a "quick drink" on an empty stomach to calm your nerves.

◆ Take medications as prescribed by your doctor. Do not stop medications just because the symptoms go away.

It usually takes six weeks to cure an ulcer, even though the symptoms may disappear in a few days. Although many drugs are available to treat ulcers these days, physicians most often prescribe cimetidine. This new drug relieves and heals ulcers, and apparently keeps them healed.

Cimetidine, which has been called a revolution in the treatment of ulcers, is an antihistamine. Histamine is well known to allergy sufferers. It can dilate capillaries, make noses run, precipitate hives, and cause other inflammatory and allergic reactions. It also stimulates stomach secretions. But cimetidine is quite different from the antihistamines used to combat allergic reactions. While conventional antihistamine drugs are incapable of counteracting gastric secretions, cimetidine essentially turns off the acid spigots in your stomach.

Before cimetidine became available, ulcer victims gobbled antacids every two hours, or took unpleasant anticholinergic medication, which slowed the formation of stomach acid, but also caused dry mouth and constipation. Anticholinergic agents were not particularly effective in reducing nocturnal acid secretions that cause pain and sleepless nights. Patients taking a single dose of oral cimetidine with a normal meal have remained free of excess digestive acids for up to eight hours. They have suffered less pain day and night, and have needed over five hundred percent fewer antacid tablets. Most important, their ulcers have healed, although there is evidence that they return once medication is discontinued. Cimetidine has caused no major side effects to date. However, the drug is not advised for pregnant women, nursing mothers, or children. It has also been found to decrease male sperm counts.

Cimetidine is used to treat other disorders, including the Zollinger-Ellison syndrome, a disease which combines hard-to-cure peptic ulcers, massive secretion of stomach acid, and tumors of the pancreas. In the past, the only treatment for the syndrome was total gastrectomy (removal of the stomach). Now it can be treated with cimetidine and other forms of medical therapy.

Recent medical reports indicate that cimetidine is so successful that doctors are prescribing it for a far greater variety of conditions than the clinical uses for which the Food and Drug Administration (FDA) approved it in 1977. Of 2,840 patients receiving cimetidine in one hospital study, less than ten percent received it for FDA-approved uses, and only twenty percent had documented peptic disease of any sort. The rest were given cimetidine for gastritis, gastrointestinal bleeding, and undiagnosed abdominal pain, and, as mentioned earlier, esophagitis. After noticing that nationwide sales of cimetidine amount to $500 million annually, the investigators became curious about how it is actually used in clinical practice. They reported that physicians use drugs for "investigational" purposes other than those approved by the FDA about ten percent of the time. If this study is any indication, cimetidine is prescribed for unapproved uses far more often than other drugs. In 1980, cimetidine, marketed under the brand name Tagamet, was the top-selling prescription drug in the United States, supplanting the tranquilizer Valium. The reason for this popularity is that ulcer patients treated with this drug are less likely to need surgery than in previous years.

Although other drugs have been virtually eclipsed by cimetidine, many are effective against ulcers. Promising new ulcer drugs that are still in the experimental stage include a family of prostaglandin compounds (hormonelike substances found in almost every human cell), a licorice extract called carbenoxalene, bismuth, and sucralfate, a drug derived from sucrose. Preliminary studies show sucralfate, also known as

Carafate, to be cimetidine's equal for short-term treatment of duodenal ulcer. Sucralfate has been sold in Canada since the summer of 1980, and was approved in late 1981 by the FDA for marketing and sale in the United States. Ulcer treatment has advanced on other fronts as well. Research scientists have discovered a genetic "marker" — a digestive enzyme called pepsinogen one — that is inherited and may be used to detect ulcer-prone people. Patients with duodenal ulcers tend to have abnormally high levels of this enzyme in their blood. Today, a simple blood test can be used to identify an ulcer patient's relatives who may be susceptible to duodenal ulcers. Another development involves flexible tubes called endoscopes that can be inserted through the mouth into the stomach. This allows a doctor to look at an ulcer and treat it directly, sometimes with a clotting substance or plasticlike coating that makes the ulcer stop bleeding. Laser beams are also used to cauterize ulcers (see Chapter 13). As a last resort, surgery may be necessary, especially if the ulcer is perforated or bleeding uncontrollably. In the past, surgeons removed the lower part of the stomach to relieve recurrent upper gastrointestinal bleeding, or they cut the vagus nerve, which connects the surface of the stomach with the brain and, among other functions, stimulates digestive acid. Today the trend is toward severing only those fibers in the vagus nerve that are directly responsible for acid secretion.

Occasionally, an ulcer will eat its way through the wall of the stomach or duodenum, and cause pain and infection throughout the abdomen. That is what happened to Napoleon. But more often, as in the case of Mary Queen of Scots, ulcers tend to heal themselves, no matter what you do.

If your ulcer is in the duodenum, you need not worry that it is cancerous. However, about five to ten percent of gastric ulcers turn out to be malignant and must be treated by surgery — the sooner the better. But once an ulcer, either duodenal or gastric, is diagnosed as noncancerous, medical evidence suggests that it will not become malignant. "Cancers ulcerate," the saying goes, "but ulcers don't cancerate!" However, other complications may develop. Muscle spasm or scar tissue from the ulcer may obstruct the outlet from the stomach to the duodenum, making surgery necessary. Or the ulcer may dig so deep that there is bleeding, or, less often, perforation, as the ulcer eats its way through the wall of the stomach or duodenum.

Although ulcer treatments and the outlook for better detection have improved, major problems remain. Physicians can heal ulcers, but cannot *keep* them healed. From seventy-five to eighty percent of those persons who develop one ulcer get at least one more, probably because whatever caused the first ulcer is still a factor. Whence comes yet another medical saying, "Once an ulcer, always an ulcer!"

Perhaps the best advice for people with ulcers is to stop smoking, stop worrying, and figure out what part of your lifestyle and diet might be causing or aggravating the problem. In his book *Clinical Gastroenterology*, Dr. Howard M. Spiro urges his gastroenterologist colleagues and their patients to understand that ". . . an ulcer is only a minor annoyance. It is not a tragedy, neither a castrophe nor a burden, but merely a small reminder of mortality."

Cirrhosis of the Liver

Question: what is about the size of a football, hovers above your stomach, and is even more mistreated than that organ? *Answer:* the liver, your body's chemical laboratory where at least five thousand biochemical reactions take place. Among other services, this workhorse produces quick energy when you need it, regulates blood sugar, manufactures new body proteins and more than one thousand different enzymes, stores certain vitamins and minerals, produces blood clotting factors, and sends forth a pint of bile a day, without which you could not digest a single raisin. Bile, a yellowish orange fluid, which resembles car motor oil, helps your body digest fats. Two-thirds of the liver's blood supply first circulates through your stomach, pancreas, and intestines. The liver must then clean that blood, balance the chemicals therein, detoxify poisons, and in many other ways, deal with the food you eat. The liver can transform many substances — even gasoline — into water-soluble compounds. And when you drink too much alcohol, your liver, ever accommodating, similarly transforms those devilish spirits and prevents them from accumulating in your blood, brain, and other body tissues. The liver can even regenerate new tissue when its own is damaged.

But there are limits. When you drink too much alcohol, fat accumulates in your liver. The question is, how much is too much? By one definition, a heavy drinker is someone who drinks more alcohol than his doctor. Obviously, the amount varies from individual to individual. The more you drink, the fatter your liver becomes. Stop drinking, and the fat disappears. Start drinking again, and the fat comes back. Continue the boozing, say ten to fifteen years, and the liver is likely to lose its smooth, uniform texture and take on a knobby, yellow appearance that says: cirrhosis! The liver looks this way because its cells have degenerated, died, and hardened into scar tissue that interferes with the flow of blood through the liver.

A French physician, René Theophile Hyacinthe Laennec, first described cirrhosis in the early 1800s after noticing at a series of autopsies a number of livers that were yellow, knobby, and hard. Laennec, who also invented the stethoscope, suspected that these unhealthy-looking livers might somehow be related to rum and the like. A medical text published in 1802 declares that the most common cause of "scirrhous livers" is intemperate use of "spirituous liquors." In the 1930s, research scientists began to suspect that poor nutrition was to blame. Studies in the 1940s suggested that even small amounts of alcohol — so-called social drinking — could cause accumulations of fat or "fatty liver," a common prelude to cirrhosis. In the 1960s, scientists tried to learn what causes cirrhosis by studying rats. However, the rats refused to drink enough alcohol to seriously damage their livers!

Science next turned to baboons. In one study, fifteen were fed a balanced diet plus the human equivalent of a quart of whiskey daily for four years. All the baboons developed fatty livers, five progressed to alcoholic hepatitis (an inflammation of the liver also related to alcohol abuse), and two developed cirrhosis.

These studies proved that alcohol by itself can cause

cirrhosis. But light drinkers and teetotalers get it too. Some skeptics say that overdoses of *anything* — whether alcohol, carrot juice, or milk — will damage the body. The force-feeding of grain to geese to fatten their livers for paté de fois gras is a case in point. The effect of nutrition on cirrhosis is also unclear. Though many alcoholics with cirrhosis are malnourished, the disease also occurs among those who are well nourished. Apparently, feeding nutritious food to alcoholics does not help to prevent cirrhosis.

Today it is known that numerous conditions can lead to cirrhosis, and that alcoholism, though by far the most common, is only one of them. Cirrhosis may occur as a result of several types of viral hepatitis (to be discussed next), severe drug reactions, prolonged exposure to environmental toxins, prolonged obstruction of the bile ducts, some forms of heart disease, certain parasitic conditions, and a number of abnormalities in the way the body handles copper, iron, and other chemicals.

Thus, much information about cirrhosis of the liver remains inconclusive. Not all alcoholics develop cirrhosis. It usually strikes people in their forties and fifties, but teenagers can develop it too, and twice as many men as women die from the disease. In the United States, cirrhosis is the third or fourth leading cause of death among adults. It is a legendary ailment among the French. Their *crises de foie* (liver attacks), said to be the country's most common ailment, have sent many a Frenchman to Vichy to partake of the healing mineral waters.

Nobody knows how much alcohol it takes to produce cirrhosis. The length of time you drink appears to have a greater effect than the amount. Heavy drinking for as little as two days has been known to increase liver fat and cell damage in a small number of highly susceptible people. The consumption of four to five drinks daily for several weeks is likely to cause fat to accumulate in the liver. But cirrhosis usually develops only after a decade or more of heavy boozing. Some experts believe that people who drink one or two martinis, or the equivalent, daily can damage their livers. But the American Liver Foundation (ALF), a private voluntary health agency, says that one or two drinks of hard liquor (or its equivalent) daily appears to be a safe level of drinking for most people. The ALF defines heavy drinking as one-half to one pint, or eight to sixteen ounces of hard liquor daily. Even if one hundred drinkers drink that much every day for fifteen years or more, only one-third will develop cirrhosis, another third will develop fatty livers, and the remainder will have only minor liver problems. Cause for celebration? Hardly. Consider the odds before you pop another champagne cork.

The early damage of cirrhosis is silent. After awhile you begin to lose weight, suffer stomach upsets, and vomit. You cannot digest fats. Often your doctor is the first to detect your fatty liver during a physical examination. Sometimes it veritably bulges from the right side of your abdomen. Blood tests or a liver biopsy — in which your physician draws a piece of liver tissue about the size of a two-inch automatic pencil lead through a needle inserted into the abdomen — can confirm the degree of damage. If it is extensive, the cells of your liver, laden with fat, refuse to help your body digest food. Bile backs into your bloodstream, yellowing your skin and eyes. The bile backup may cause your skin to itch. Spidery blood vessels may appear on your face and neck. Your belly swells from fluid accumulations caused by blood unable to flow through your liver. You may vomit blood. Your palms turn red, your blood refuses to clot. If you are male, as most cirrhotics are, your breasts may enlarge and irreversible impotence may occur.

Scared? Sit down. You need another drink. Better yet, you need to quit. The scarring of your liver cannot be reversed, but it can be slowed down or even stopped. All it takes is quitting the booze. Sixty percent of all cirrhotics who stop drinking are alive and well five years later. Close to one hundred percent of those who don't stop are dead five years later, or near-dead from hemorrhage or liver failure.

When cirrhosis is caused by other factors, such as hepatitis, your physician may recommend treatment with corticosteroid drugs, or with certain antiviral compounds. In some cases, cirrhosis caused by hepatitis is treated with interferon, a biological response modifier that improves the body's ability to fend off viral infection, and may eradicate the virus in some cases.

Vaccines are under development to prevent infections that may lead to cirrhosis, and research scientists are trying to discover better ways to detect and treat cirrhosis and its complications. These include abdominal swelling, bleeding from internal varicose veins (varices) in the esophagus, the development of scar tissue after liver cell damage, and coma.

Hundreds of liver transplants have been performed in the United States since the mid-1960s, but survival times are no cause for celebration. Until recently, less than half of those who received transplants could hope to live even a year. A substantially higher survival rate — at least in the short run — has recently been reported by Dr. Thomas E. Starzl of the University of Pittsburgh School of Medicine, the man who performed the first liver transplant in 1964. According to an article in the July 30, 1981 *New England Journal of Medicine*, ten out of twelve patients in his study were still alive an average of one year after their operations. They had received an experimental drug, cyclosporin A, that suppresses the body's immune system so it will not attack the transplanted liver. But even if cyclosporin A proves effective in the long run, liver transplants are not likely to become routine because the procedure itself is difficult to perform even if the body accepts the new organ. An "artificial liver" currently under development supports patients only for very short periods of time. This suggests that until medical science can cure liver disease — and that will not be soon — you would do well to prevent it. Cutting down on excess boozing is the best way.

You should also learn to recognize the symptoms of liver disease, whether caused by cirrhosis, hepatitis, or some less common disorder:

◆ Jaundice (yellowed skin and whites of the eyes). This is often the first, and sometimes the *only*, sign of liver disease.
◆ Very dark-colored urine, which usually appears before jaundice.
◆ Gray, yellow, or light-colored stools.

◆ Nausea, vomiting, and / or loss of appetite.
◆ Vomiting blood or passing it in the stools, either of which indicates intestinal bleeding.
◆ Abdominal pain and swelling, the latter caused by an accumulation of fluid in the abdominal cavity.
◆ Prolonged itching all over the body, caused by jaundice.
◆ A five percent loss or gain in weight within two months.
◆ Fatigue or loss of stamina.
◆ Loss of sexual drive or performance.
◆ Sleep disturbances, mental confusion, and coma. These occur when poisonous substances that the liver can no longer detoxify reach the brain.

The health of your liver is determined by the substances to which you expose it. To preserve this indispensable organ, drink in moderation, if you must drink at all, do not mix alcohol with drugs, avoid unnecessary medications, and never mix prescription drugs without consulting your doctor. Excess amounts of vitamin A and niacin, and very large doses of other vitamins can harm your liver. The recently publicized liquid protein diets are another form of assault not only on the liver, but upon the heart and kidneys as well. There are far safer ways to lose weight.

Twentieth-century livers must also withstand environmental pollutants and other chemicals that you cannot avoid. Fifty, even twenty-five, years ago the liver was not confronted with the variety of toxins it faces today. Our ancestors did not assault their livers with aerosol sprays. Automobile pollution was unknown. When using chemicals at home, work, or in your garden, the American Liver Foundation recommends that you:

◆ Make sure there is good ventilation.
◆ Follow directions on the label.
◆ Never mix chemical products.
◆ Don't get chemicals on your skin. They can be absorbed, so wash off promptly if you are exposed.
◆ Do not inhale chemicals, and wear protective clothing when using them.

Your liver is the one organ in your digestive system that you cannot do without. Your esophagus can be bypassed, and your stomach, gallbladder, pancreas, all of your large, and some of your small, intestine can be removed. But when your liver goes, you go with it.

Hepatitis

The other major liver disease is hepatitis, or inflammation of the liver. Fortunately, hepatitis is not as serious as it sounds: almost everybody who gets it recovers. Perhaps the most serious aspect of hepatitis is the alarming rate at which the disease is increasing. About one million Americans are afflicted annually — half of them children — and about eight hundred thousand people in the United States carry hepatitis B or hepatitis non-A, non-B virus in their bodies. The World Health Organization estimates that there are one hundred million hepatitis "carriers" throughout the world. These carriers are not themselves ill, but can pass the disease on to you or your family without anybody being aware of it.

Although hepatitis usually is caused by viruses, other substances such as alcohol, certain drugs, and chemicals in the environment can cause it too. At least three different types of viral hepatitis have been identified: hepatitis A, formerly called infectious hepatitis; hepatitis B, formerly called serum hepatitis; and, for lack of a better name, non-A, non-B hepatitis. The last is caused by one or more viruses that, when scientists eventually identify them, will probably be called hepatitis C, D, and E.

Hepatitis A is a highly contagious disease that primarily afflicts children and young adults. The liver becomes tender and enlarged. Symptoms usually begin with pain in the upper right side, nausea, weakness, loss of appetite, headache, and flulike fever. Sometimes these symptoms are so mild that they are dismissed as a case of flu or grippe. In more serious cases, victims may develop profound fatigue, pain, and tenderness in the upper right side. Occasionally, in very severe cases, jaundice develops, making your skin and the whites of your eyes appear yellow, and turning urine orangish brown. Most of these symptoms usually disappear in about two weeks. But the fatigue may last for weeks or months. There is no cure for hepatitis other than rest and the passage of time. Fortunately, hepatitis A infection rarely causes lasting liver damage or leads to more serious liver disease. Most important, it is preventable.

The hepatitis A virus is excreted in feces and is spread by direct contact with an infected person's feces, or by indirect contamination of fingers or eating utensils and dishes. Water or food — including raw or steamed clams, oysters, and mussels — may also be contaminated by hepatitis A virus. This disease prevails in areas with poor sanitary facilities, and in crowded places like day-care centers, mental hospitals, and military camps. From the Crusades to Vietnam, hepatitis has felled many a fighting man. By the time anybody discovers what is happening, an epidemic may have started. Hepatitis A also occurs more frequently among homosexual than among heterosexual men, and has recently been identified as one of the infections — in addition to the diarrheal disorder known as the "gay bowel syndrome" — that appears to be sexually transmitted. Transmission can also occur among heterosexual men and women who engage in oral-anal contact or anal intercourse.

It is often possible to protect people who have already been exposed to hepatitis A with an injection of immune serum globulin, a blood protein rich in antibodies that helps provide immunity for three to four months. The sooner this injection is given after exposure, the better. These shots are also strongly recommended for travelers to countries where sanitation is poor.

A vaccine to prevent hepatitis A is also under development, but will not be ready for testing in humans for many years. Meanwhile, the best way to prevent this disease is good sanitation — avoiding potentially contaminated food and water, and meticulous handwashing after going to the bathroom and before eating meals. You also should avoid intimate physical contact with infected people, with their body fluids, and with their food and eating utensils.

Hepatitis B is a far more serious infection because it can lead to lingering liver inflammation (chronic hepatitis), and may be associated with cirrhosis of the liver and primary liver cancer. However, complications occur only in about five percent of all cases. More important, about ten percent of the people who contract hepatitis B become carriers thereafter. They don't necessarily show signs of infection themselves, but they are capable of passing the disease on to others.

The hepatitis B virus is transmitted through blood and other body fluids such as breast milk, saliva, and semen. A pregnant woman can transmit the virus to her baby. Transmission can also take place by blood transfusion, mouth-to-mouth or other sexual contact, or by injecting the skin with contaminated needles during ear piercing, tattooing, acupuncture, and dental and medical procedures. There have been reports that the disease can spread via cuts caused by computer cards. Among those who become infected are users of illicit drugs, blood bank and hospital workers, and medical professionals (even though carriers can be identified by a blood test). Male homosexuals as a group have an incidence of hepatitis B more than ten times that of the general population.

Symptoms of hepatitis B are similar to those of hepatitis A — fatigue, nausea, jaundice, and dark urine. In hepatitis B, however, these symptoms are more severe and last up to six months instead of six weeks. Injections with hepatitis B immune globulin (HBIG) may help prevent hepatitis B infections in people who have been exposed, but this serum is very expensive and must be administered before the disease actually occurs. HBIG also appears to keep newborn infants whose mothers are hepatitis B carriers from themselves becoming lifelong carriers.

More recently, research scientists have developed, and the FDA has licensed, a hepatitis B vaccine that is made from a virus taken from the blood plasma of people who are chronic hepatitis B carriers. The vaccine, when tested in a clinical study involving 1,083 male homosexuals, reduced the incidence of hepatitis B by more than ninety percent, and caused few side effects. While inoculation against hepatitis B is not practical or necessary for the general population, people whose lifestyles or jobs expose them to the disease now have reliable protection. The importance of the vaccine to doctors and dentists is incalculable, for if they become hepatitis B carriers, they could be barred from practicing medicine. This happened to a dentist in Baltimore, Maryland who, as a carrier, was transmitting hepatitis B to his patients.

People who are known carriers of hepatitis B infection should:

◆ Never share any items that may puncture the skin or become contaminated with body fluids. These include razor blades, scissors, nail files, needles, toothbrushes, and enema or douche equipment.
◆ Never donate blood.
◆ Abstain from kissing and sexual contact during the acute stage of the disease.
◆ Cover cuts and sores to avoid exposing others.
◆ Tell your doctor and dentist, laboratory technicians, and others who may draw blood or perform surgical procedures about your disease.
◆ Tell family members and other intimates to see a physician.

Like hepatitis B, a third type of hepatitis called non-A, non-B (NANB) can develop into chronic disease, and is often spread by blood transfusion. Each year an estimated one hundred thousand to one hundred-fifty thousand people contract chemically detectable posttransfusion hepatitis, about ninety percent of it the NANB type. The agent that causes it has not been identified. Indeed, this form of hepatitis was recognized only after donor blood that was found free of hepatitis B virus nevertheless caused hepatitis several months after transfusion.

No blood test yet can detect NANB carriers, although there are indirect testing methods. One of these uses the level of alanine aminotransferase (ALT), an enzyme manufactured in the liver, as an indicator of NANB hepatitis. The theory is that people with hepatitis have some degree of liver damage, and therefore have elevated concentrations of liver enzymes such as ALT. Meanwhile, NANB hepatitis carriers continue to be discovered mainly when blood they donate infects a recipient. Despite the lack of detection methods, the rate of hepatitis has been cut by nearly two-thirds by eliminating the use of blood from paid, commercial donors, and using only volunteer blood. A vaccine for NANB hepatitis cannot be developed until the virus or viruses that cause it are identified.

About two to four percent of people who have had hepatitis B, and forty to fifty percent of those who have had NANB infections, can develop chronic or persistent hepatitis that continues for decades. Chronic hepatitis may be caused by alcohol, the most potent tranquilizers, certain antibiotics and "sulfa" drugs, halothane anesthesia, insecticides, industrial solvents, and metallic compounds containing arsenic, iron, mercury, and gold, all of which can cause liver inflammation. A few patients with chronic hepatitis appear to have defects in the immune system that normally defends the liver against disease.

Although symptoms of chronic hepatitis are usually milder than those of acute hepatitis, the continuing inflammation can permanently scar the liver, and lead to cirrhosis or irreversible liver failure. In cases where this seems likely, your physician may recommend that you take cortisonelike drugs. These steroids are particularly effective against chronic hepatitis that is unrelated to viral infection.

Gallbladder Disease

You may be one of the sixteen to twenty million Americans with a miniature stone quarry in your gut. It may contain one gallstone or one hundred or, in rare cases, gallstones by the thousands. Gallstones are not really "stones" but clumps of fat (cholesterol) or bile-pigment deposits that collect in the gallbladder and form stones. They range in size from smaller than a pinhead to larger than an egg, and come in shades of white, yellow, tan, or black. Gallstones may be round or egg-shaped and, if several gallstones lie close together, their sides may be flattened by the pressure of their neighbors, resulting in multifaceted gallstones.

The typical gallstone patient has four outstanding characteristics, known in medical circles as the four Fs:

- Fat.
- Fecund.
- Female.
- Forty.

Gallstones tend to afflict overweight women over age forty who have had several children. Although even teenagers develop gallstones, once you turn forty, the chances of having them jump from one in ten to one in five. The stone-prone include people who are pregnant, obese, chronically anemic, those who have Crohn's disease or various metabolic illnesses, and those who take oral contraceptives, estrogen, or a number of other drugs. Although the causes of gallstones are not well understood, the incidence of gallstones is known to vary with race and geography. About seventy-three percent of American Indian women and fifty-seven percent of Swedish women have gallstones, while stones seldom occur among Orientals and Africans. So-called pigment gallstones, which are formed primarily from bile pigments, are very common in some areas of Asia, but are far less common in the United States.

About half of the people who have gallstones never even know it. Their gallstones are "silent" because they produce no symptoms. The other half, however, develop "gallbladder trouble" — more formally known as biliary tract disease.

The source of all this trouble is the gallbladder, a two- to three-inch eggplant-shaped organ that hangs under your liver and serves as a temporary storehouse for an ounce or two of concentrated liver bile. During digestion, the gallbladder releases this substance through the bile ducts and into the duodenum where it helps to digest fats. An estimated eighty to ninety percent of all gallstones that occur in Americans form when bile contains too much cholesterol. Thus, gallstones are actually a liver disease since it is the liver that secretes the abnormal bile.

Cholesterol, a fat which ordinarily cannot be dissolved in water, is dissolved in bile by the detergentlike action of bile salts. However, if too much cholesterol is present in bile, it cannot be held in solution, just as too much sugar in iced tea drops to the bottom of the glass. The cholesterol makes small crystals that grow to form gallstones. Thus, people who are obese or those who take oral contraceptives, estrogens, or certain other drugs are more likely to develop gallstones because they tend to secrete high levels of cholesterol.

While gallstones may lie quietly in the gallbladder, sometimes, for unknown reasons, they migrate from your gallbladder and get stuck in the narrow ducts leading to the duodenum. When this happens, bile cannot flow freely into the intestine. You may feel faintness, nausea, chills, indigestion, or pain that resembles a stitch in the side. Or you may suffer severe, knifelike pain in the upper right side of your abdomen, which spreads to your back or right shoulder. The pain can be so intense that you vomit, become wet with perspiration, and perhaps develop fever and chills. This usually happens within one to two hours after eating a rich, fatty meal. If you experience these symptoms, call a doctor right away. Your gallbladder attack (known as acute cholecystitis) may be over in a few minutes, or it may last a week, subsiding only when the stone drops back into your gallbladder or moves into your intestine.

If a gallstone permanently lodges in your cystic duct — or, worse, your common bile duct — it will prevent liver bile from reaching your intestine. A blocked bile duct can cause painful inflammation of the gallbladder or distention of the duct itself. Blockage can also cause infection of the ducts, and / or jaundice. Your stools may turn light gray or white because bile, the substance that turns your stools dark, is prevented from reaching your intestines. And your urine may turn the color of tea or cola because some of the substances in bile back up into the blood stream and are excreted in urine. If any of these symptoms occur, don't wait to see your doctor; go straight to a hospital emergency room.

Some cases of gallbladder trouble respond to medical treatment, but the usual cure for these attacks is removal of the gallbladder. The first such operation was performed in 1867 on Mary Wiggins Burnsworth of McCordsville, Indiana. Surgery was a risky business in those days. There were no surgical hospitals, no operating rooms, and no trained nurses. Indeed, anyone who submitted to abdominal surgery accepted a greater risk than astronauts who are sent into space today. Mary Wiggins Burnsworth was a tailoress who at age twenty-seven felt an enlargement about the size of a hickory nut in the lower part of her abdomen. Food, drink, and exercise triggered bouts of pain lasting three to four hours. The enlargement grew until she could not walk. Finally, she could not even operate her sewing machine, and was forced to give up her job. A tender mass filled the right side of her abdomen. Several physicians thought she had an ovarian tumor, but a surgeon named Dr. John S. Bobbs decided that the tumor had nothing to do with her female organs. Because he was unsure of its true nature, he was reluctant to recommend an operation. It was Mary herself who insisted on surgery, for she wanted something done to relieve her pain.

Thus, on June 15, 1867, Mary, Dr. Bobbs, seven other doctors, and a medical student met on the third floor of a building that housed a wholesale drugstore on the lower floors. The doctors proceeded to prepare Mary for surgery by anesthetizing her with chloroform. Dr. Bobbs began his incision in the lower abdomen, then extended it upward. Before long, he came upon a large, translucent mass, which he did not at first recognize as a greatly distended gallbladder. Then, as he cut through the thin wall, an enormous number of gallstones shot out with great force. He removed still more stones with his finger, although one remained so tightly lodged he could not budge it. Once the sac had been emptied, he sewed it up, and later described the procedure as the first "lithotomy" of the gallbladder. It was, in fact, the first surgical procedure of any kind upon that organ.

Mary survived the operation and lived another forty-six years. Dr. Bobbs lived another three. Some time later, when the medical world recognized the significance of the surgery she had undergone, Mary Wiggins Burnsworth was asked to appear at the 1905 annual meeting of the American Medical Association to attend an exhibit commemorating Dr. Bobbs's contribution to surgery and medicine.

Today, gallbladder surgery — called cholecystectomy — is one of the most frequently performed operations in the United States. About half a million cholecystectomies are performed each year, at no small cost to the patient. In

1981, a single procedure in Fairfax County, Virginia, cost about $5,400, broken down as follows:

Surgeon's fee	$1,055.00
Anesthesia	374.00
X rays	179.00
Hospital	3,746.03
T O T A L	$5,354.03

A nine-day stay in the hospital, in turn, cost this patient $1,260 for a semiprivate room and nursing care, $540 for the use of the operating room for 2½ hours, $314 for lab fees, $240 for surgical supplies, and $110 for the use of the emergency room.

In more than the profit-making sense, cholecystectomy is a highly successful procedure since it cures eighty-five percent of all gallbladder disorders. Although the operation is generally safe, five to eight thousand patients die each year as a result of the surgery. The patients who undergo this procedure are often elderly, and sometimes are poor surgical risks as well.

In general, however, people whose gallbladders have been removed do very well without them. Their livers take over the gallbladder's job, and secrete bile directly into the intestine. Some animals with digestive systems much like those of humans don't even have gallbladders, which suggests that nature may be trying to tell us something.

Sometimes surgery is recommended for young people with silent gallstones because they are likely to cause trouble as a person grows older. Conservative physicians, however, do not advocate such radical treatment for something that is not yet causing trouble and — in the case of older patients — may never cause trouble.

Gallstones are seldom life-threatening unless the gallbladder's tissues have been destroyed, or a stone has worn through the gallbladder wall or through one of the ducts, and has caused peritonitis throughout the abdominal cavity. Stones that block the flow of bile endanger the liver itself, and could be fatal. However, these complications are the exception, not the rule.

Gallbladder operations are numerous because the troublesome gallbladder continues to produce stones. Thus, the first gallbladder attack is likely to lead to continuing attacks unless you take steps to correct the problem. These include changes in diet and living habits: you should cut down on fatty foods such as butter, mayonnaise, eggs, and deep-fried and gas-producing foods that seem to cause symptoms; drink lots of water; and get plenty of outdoor exercise.

The last word on surgery usually comes from the patient. Many people prefer surgery — a one-shot, if severe, solution — to less costly medical measures like giving up fatty foods. And many people who have suffered the pain of a gallbladder attack are willing to undergo surgery in order to avoid a repetition of that experience.

Gallbladder surgery may eventually become unnecessary — some critics of the medical establishment say that it already is — if scientists succeed in developing a new drug to dissolve gallstones. So far, the best known is chenodeoxycholic ("chenic") acid. Chenic acid, or CDCA, is one of the natural components of human bile. During the late 1960s, research scientists discovered that chenic acid, administered in capsules every day for one to two years, could completely dissolve or reduce the size of gallstones among half of the patients they studied. However, in the years since, chenic acid has proven to be inconsistently effective. Recently, results of the National Cooperative Gallstone Study, sponsored by the National Institute of Arthritis, Diabetes, and Digestive and Kidney Diseases, have shown that chenic acid has limited value as an alternative to surgery for patients with cholesterol gallstones. The study showed that after two years of treatment, only fourteen percent of 305 patients receiving 750 milligrams of the drug daily experienced complete dissolution of gallstones, and another twenty-seven percent experienced partial dissolution. Moreover, gallbladder attacks remained as numerous and severe as they had been before treatment, and surgery was performed just as often. The Food and Drug Administration is now evaluating the results of the study and deciding whether to allow drug companies to market chenic acid for the treatment of cholesterol gallstones.

Other studies of gallstone-dissolving drugs are exploring the effects of diet in combination with ursodeoxycholic acid (UDCA). Closely related to chenic acid, this drug is also a normal constituent of bile. It has been found that smaller doses of UDCA are just as effective as chenic acid in dissolving gallstones. It is important to find a drug that dissolves gallstones successfully, not only to avoid surgery, but because some patients who undergo cholecystectomy find that cholesterol gallstones continue to form in their bile ducts.

Another possible gallstone-dissolving drug is aspirin, which is being studied in animals. For example, studies of prairie dog gallbladders seem to support the hypothesis that cholesterol gallstone growth is facilitated by certain mucus secretions in the gallbladder. Aspirin is known to inhibit mucus secretion in other organs, so the researchers measured its effect on mucus secretion in gallbladders of normal prairie dogs and of prairie dogs fed a high-cholesterol diet. The results showed that aspirin inhibited gallbladder mucus secretion in both groups of prairie dogs by twenty to eighty-five percent. These observations remain to be tested in humans.

Although gallstones have been around for a long time — they have been found in Egyptian mummies — it is still not known what causes them. The notion that fatty foods trigger gallstone attacks is no more proven than the hypothesis that overeating and poor eating habits lead to gallstones. There is epidemiological evidence that people on a high-fiber diet secrete liver bile that contains less cholesterol, and therefore, is less likely to form gallstones. Gallbladder troubles are exceedingly rare in Africa and other underdeveloped countries that have not yet converted to Western diets. During World War II when foods rich in cholesterol were not available, the incidence of gallstone problems fell dramatically among the Danish people, who were forced to give up their usual rich diets. And recent studies by Canadian researchers show that in twenty-five gallstone patients, increased consumption of fiber caused high cholesterol levels in bile to drop to normal.

◇ ◇ ◇

Pancreatitis

Pancreatitis is an inflammation or soreness of the most powerful digestive organ in your body: the pancreas gland. The size and shape of a large dog's tongue, the pancreas is about six inches long, grayish pink, and located just behind the lower part of your stomach and in front of your spine. In animals, the pancreas is called the sweetbread.

The pancreas has two jobs: it is best known for producing insulin, which keeps blood sugar at a proper level and sees that the body utilizes it properly. Diabetes, the leading disease of the pancreas, occurs when that organ does not produce enough insulin.

Each day, the pancreas also produces about two pints of pancreatic juice loaded with enzymes, which are chemical ferments needed for digestion. As food leaves your stomach and enters the duodenum, the latter starts manufacturing a hormone which prods the pancreas into production. Pancreatic juices not only aid in the digestion of proteins, starches, and fats, but also — because of their alkaline content — neutralize acidic gastric juices and prevent them from eating away the tender tissues of the small intestine.

Pancreatitis, the major digestive disease of the pancreas, has many causes: injury during surgery on a nearby organ, nutritional deficiencies, prolonged use of certain drugs, cigarette smoking, pregnancy, disturbances of fat metabolism, and intestinal abnormalities. But the two biggest causes of pancreatitis are years of heavy alcohol consumption and gallstones. Poor plumbing adds to the problem. The pancreas shares with the liver and gallbladder a common exit duct into the duodenum. Thus, if a gallstone blocks a duct, it will also block the release of pancreatic juice into the intestine. Large amounts of alcohol are suspected to cause swelling and spasm in the duct that leads to the duodenum. In addition, alcohol causes the pancreas to secrete too much pancreatic juice, possibly because alcohol is such a powerful stimulant of stomach acid. Scientists suspect that stomach acid, in turn, stimulates the pancreas to oversecrete enzymes that damage the pancreas. This combination of events, in effect, causes the pancreas to "blow up" as its digestive enzymes, prevented from reaching the intestine, proceed to digest and destroy the pancreas itself.

Acute pancreatitis is a medical emergency. It causes excruciating abdominal pains just above or around your navel. The pain may radiate to your back and hurt even more if you move or press on your abdomen. The pain becomes worse when you eat a meal, and is usually accompanied by nausea and vomiting, constipation, jaundice, and rapid pulse rate. In very severe cases, the pancreas may hemorrhage, resulting in shock.

Pancreatitis must be treated in the hospital, where your doctor will try to give your pancreas a rest by stopping the secretion of pancreatic juice. This means no food or liquids by mouth, a tube in your stomach to remove gastric secretions and relieve pain and nausea, intravenous fluids, and drugs that inhibit pain and pancreatic secretion. Surgery is seldom necessary. After you recover, your doctor will determine whether gallstones have caused pancreatitis and treat or remove them. If alcohol is at the root of the problem — and a substantial percentage of alcoholics develop pancreatitis — you must stop drinking. The pancreas has exceptional ability to regenerate itself, but there are limits.

To prevent further attacks, your doctor will probably recommend a low-fat diet, frequent snacks which do not overstimulate the pancreas, and drug therapy. Excessive food or alcohol consumption could trigger another attack, but one drink a day probably will not hurt. However, many alcoholics will not give up their cocktails at any price — even when their lives are at stake.

Chronic pancreatitis afflicts about twenty thousand to fifty thousand people in the United States, mostly men between the ages of thirty and fifty. This recurring form of the disease can gradually destroy the tissues of your pancreas. First come the increasingly frequent attacks of abdominal pain, then weight loss and diarrhea, followed by permanent damage to your pancreas, including impaired digestion and diabetes that is irreversible because the pancreas can no longer produce insulin. Occasionally, there are no clear symptoms of pancreatitis, either acute or chronic, and the condition may go undetected until damage is irreversible.

Although surgery is seldom needed for acute pancreatitis, cysts sometimes develop because of the inflammation, and may have to be removed surgically. If gallbladder disease is the cause of pancreatitis, a surgeon will remove the gallstones blocking the pancreatic duct. Sometimes surgery is the only way to relieve severe pain caused by chronic pancreatitis, although, for most cases, surgery is not recommended.

In a procedure called a subtotal pancreatectomy, a surgeon removes all but about an inch off one end of the pancreas, and attaches the remainder to a loop of intestine. Or the pancreas can be split lengthwise and attached to the small intestine. Both procedures allow dammed-up pancreatic juice to flow freely into the intestine, and relieve pain caused by the pressures of blockage. As a last resort, the entire pancreas can be removed in a procedure called total pancreatectomy. At one time, this meant certain death. Today, while the procedure will shorten your life expectancy, doctors can prescribe substitute enzymes that will keep you alive — if uncomfortable — plus medications and diet to control diabetes that develops when most or all of the pancreas is removed. Actor Peter O'Toole has had this procedure.

The role that emotions play in causing pancreatitis is controversial. Some digestive disease experts downplay stress as a cause of pancreatitis, and say only that it can make the disease worse once it is established. Others, however, acknowledge that worry and aggravation can excite the vagus nerve, which causes the stomach to produce excess hydrochloric acid. The acid, in turn, is a powerful stimulator of pancreatic secretion. People with pancreatitis who continue to consume alcohol eventually kill themselves. They know they should stop drinking, yet do. Who is to say this refusal to preserve their own lives is not — in some profound way — an emotional problem?

CHAPTER 10

The Lower Depths

JOHN HARVEY KELLOGG of *Colon Hygiene* fame once wrote that the lower intestine is the source of more disease and physical suffering than any other part of the body. He was referring to the clogged or constipated colon that had been poisoned by its own "seething mass of putrefying food residues." Kellogg's theory of "autointoxication" never won much acceptance in medical circles, partly because his methods of treatment were so far out.

The kinds of colon distress doctors see today are known to have far more complex causes. These diseases include ileitis, or Crohn's disease, and — moving ever lower — ulcerative colitis, irritable bowel syndrome, appendicitis, diverticular disease, and hemorrhoids.

Inflammatory bowel diseases — which include ileitis and ulcerative colitis — are the most serious and perplexing of the intestinal disorders. These diseases, along with irritable bowel syndrome, which will be discussed later, are the humiliating "bathroom" diseases about which people are so unwilling to talk, for they cause crampy abdominal pain, gas, and recurrent diarrhea. Inflammatory bowel diseases (IBD) are on the rise, though nobody knows why. They hit hardest at young people, generally never go away and, worst of all,

141

continue to baffle medical scientists, who have discovered neither cause nor cure for these conditions.

Ileitis, or Crohn's Disease

Because nobody knows what causes it, Crohn's disease is named after Dr. Burrill B. Crohn, who first described it in 1932. Crohn's disease, also known as ileitis, is a severe and chronic inflammation of the deeper layers of the intestinal wall. It usually involves the ileum or lower section of the small intestine, but may occur in any part of the intestine, including the colon. If it affects one or more segments of the small intestine, it is called regional enteritis. To add to the confusion, it has other names as well: granulomatous colitis, colitis, ileocolitis, cicatrizing enterocolitis, and terminal ileitis. One woman, when told that she had terminal ileitis, almost fainted from the shock until her doctor explained that "terminal" referred to the location of the inflammation at the far end of her small intestine, and not to the odds on whether she would survive!

This disease afflicts more than ten thousand Americans, primarily young people. Many Jewish people develop Crohn's disease. It usually strikes before age thirty and, for unknown reasons, appears to be occurring at increasingly early ages. Generally, the younger the victim, the more severe the disease.

Crohn's disease often causes a narrowing of the passageway through the small intestine which, in turn, causes severe abdominal pain, usually in the lower right side. Diarrhea may occur up to twenty times a day, and is often accompanied by blood, pus, and large amounts of mucus. Frequently, this severe diarrhea causes anal fissures or lesions. The skin around the anus may split or ulcerate. Fistulas (abnormal passages between loops of intestine and other internal organs) occur because the inflammation caused by Crohn's disease is so deep that the usually smooth outer surface of the intestine becomes rough and sticks to neighboring structures. The inflammation may affect the adjoining area and burrow tunnels into the vulva, vagina, scrotum, or bladder, requiring repeated surgery. Crohn's disease, when it is severe enough and lasts long enough, can also lead to varying degrees of malnutrition.

Beyond the intestinal tract, Crohn's disease may cause other complications including liver disorders, arthritis, skin and mucous-membrane disorders, eye lesions, urinary tract infections, and kidney stones. When ileitis occurs during childhood or early adolescence, it causes malnutrition, stunts growth, and may delay sexual development. A fourteen-year-old boy with ileitis may be trapped in a body that tires easily, stands barely four feet tall, and must be nourished by intravenous feeding.

Because Crohn's disease develops slowly, one boy suffered for two years before doctors recognized his symptoms. By then, he had diarrhea ten to twelve times a day and steadily lost weight until, at age twelve, he weighed forty-seven pounds. Another boy, at age seventeen, weighed seventy-five pounds, measured four feet, eight inches, had a bone age of twelve years, and showed no signs of puberty. Many cases of inflammatory bowel disease are not recognized for years and, sometimes, are never properly diagnosed. In other cases, growth failure may precede by years other evidence of inflammatory bowel diseases in children. But if the disease is discovered in time, and metabolic and nutritional deficiencies are remedied, the child's growth and sexual maturation will resume.

A physician's treatment of Crohn's disease consists mainly of controlling symptoms such as pain and bowel motility with antiinflammatory drugs such as sulfasalazine (commercially known as Azulfidine), corticosteroids, and sometimes immunosuppressant drugs taken by mouth or by injection. While these drugs may relieve symptoms, they do not prevent or cure attacks of ileitis, and often cause undesirable side effects. Prolonged use of corticosteroids, for example, can cause rounding of the face, weight gain, pain in the limbs, mood swings, acne, excessive hair growth, and weakness. Sulfa drugs help during severe attacks, and cause fewer harmful side effects. However, anti-diarrheal drugs and similar medications are intended for milder forms of diarrhea in people who are free of Crohn's disease.

Because Crohn's disease tends to recur, prolonged hospitalization and repeated surgery is often necessary. Many times, a surgeon removes a diseased portion of the small intestine, only to have ileitis later develop in the portion immediately adjacent. Some patients have been known to undergo five operations in six months. One out of every two people with Crohn's disease will eventually have surgery, usually for fistulas, abscesses, narrowing and blockage of the bowel, or some other complication. Generally, only parts of the lower end of the small intestine — the ileum — must be removed. Sometimes, part of the large intestine is also diseased and must be removed, a procedure known as an ileocolostomy. Less frequently, a healthy loop of the small intestine is spliced into the colon, and the diseased section is bypassed and left in place. This was the procedure used on President Eisenhower when he had surgery for ileitis in June 1956. Whatever procedure is used, the small intestine cannot be removed entirely because it is essential to the absorption of food.

Sometimes ileitis inexplicably subsides or goes into remission, only to recur just as inexplicably months or years later. If it does recur, the victim can only drink lots of fluids to reduce the serious risk of dehydration from diarrhea, and eat well.

There is no single "balanced" diet that helps ileitis patients, although the American Digestive Disease Society has a dietary plan for people with this disorder (see Appendix A). Many can tolerate all kinds of foods, while others do better, especially when their disease flares up, on a bland, low-fiber diet that does not overstimulate the bowel. If Crohn's disease causes narrowing of the bowel, a liquid diet may be necessary.

Good nutrition is not easy to maintain when you have a chronic disease such as ileitis, for it reduces your appetite and constantly uses up caloric energy. Even worse, the diseased small intestine is less able to absorb nutrients into your body. The severity of this problem depends upon how much of your small intestine is affected. If more than two to three feet are diseased or removed, or if the middle section — the jejunum — is inflamed, you may have a significant problem absorbing dietary fats and other nutrients. While certain foods may aggravate ileitis, there is no evidence that dietary factors in any way cause inflammatory bowel disease.

There is a high incidence of inflammatory bowel disease within families, suggesting that genetic factors probably play a role. Defects in the immune system are also suspected to cause inflammatory bowel disease. According to one theory, an undigested dietary protein, a virus, or bacterium could reach the bowel wall and, rather than be destroyed by the body's defense mechanisms, remain intact. This could trigger an inflammatory or allergic reaction in which the body ends up attacking and damaging its own tissues.

Another persistent, though controversial, belief is that stress causes inflammatory bowel diseases like ileitis. Although opponents of this theory maintain that Crohn's disease *causes* — rather than is caused by — emotional stress, there is little doubt that emotional factors can influence the course of the disease, and that acute psychological problems often immediately precede its occurrence. For example, one woman developed Crohn's disease just before she was to get married. When she rescheduled her wedding several months later, the disease again flared up. When she was finally well enough to get married, her husband, who had devoted himself entirely to helping her recover, was so weak and shaky he could hardly walk down the aisle.

This case is consistent with the observations of the English physician Dr. J. W. Paulley, who has noted that emotional disturbances and life crises tend to precede the onset of both Crohn's disease and ulcerative colitis. Crohn's disease patients, Dr. Paulley says, tend to hang on to abrasive situations, often attempting the role of peacemaker. One of Dr. Paulley's patients was a middle-aged woman who, as a child, tried to keep peace between her quarreling parents. She later allowed her daughter to live with her after the daughter had married, despite her resentment toward her son-in-law. About this time, her ileitis was at its worst. Her disease again flared up when her daughter and son-in-law went abroad and left her with two grandchildren. Later, her daughter's marriage failed, and the daughter convinced her mother to give up her job to take care of her grandchildren so the daughter could go to work. This created more resentment and another relapse. The woman later met a widower who proposed marriage, but she remained undecided because a lodger who was living in her house objected strongly. In her inability to "hurt" either of her suitors, she achieved yet another "no-win" situation. One problem with Crohn's disease patients, Dr. Paulley observed, is that they so often return to the abrasive environment that led to their illness in the first place. Unfortunately, there are few controlled studies of the psychogenic factors leading to inflammatory bowel disease. Nor have researchers learned much about the physical causes of inflammatory bowel disease, whether viral, bacterial, or immunological.

However, there has been some progress in treating ileitis. Some years ago, the National Institutes of Health sponsored a nationwide clinical trial to evaluate the relative merits of corticosteroids, sulfa drugs, and other medications for ileitis. The results, announced in 1980, showed that both prednisone (an adrenal hormone, or corticosteroid drug) and sulfasalazine (an antiinflammatory drug) are of value in putting active Crohn's disease into an inactive state known as remission. Sulfasalazine was found to be more effective for initial treatment of Crohn's disease, and relatively less likely to cause side effects. But prednisone was more effective for treating moderate and more severe cases of ileitis. Other investigators have found that the antimicrobial drug metronidazole, as well as immunosuppressive drugs, are effective against advanced Crohn's disease. Research scientists are trying to develop new ways to diagnose Crohn's disease, new drugs to treat it, and a vaccine to prevent it.

Ulcerative Colitis

The second, and by far the most prevalent, form of inflammatory bowel disease is ulcerative colitis. Like Crohn's disease, it goes by so many names that sometimes even doctors are not sure whether to call it colitis, chronic ulcerative colitis, idiopathic ulcerative colitis, indeterminate ulcerative colitis, primary ulcerative colitis, colitis ulcerosa, or thromboulcerative colitis. Sometimes ulcerative colitis is called "spastic colon," which is a term more correctly applied to an emotionally induced colon disorder known as irritable bowel syndrome (see next section).

Persons with ulcerative colitis have an actual inflammation of the inner lining of the large intestine. They also may have open sores in the colon that resemble ulcers in the stomach or duodenum, painful abdominal cramps, high fever, gas, and bloody diarrhea that occurs up to two dozen times a day and lasts from weeks to years. Bouts of ulcerative colitis sometimes subside, only to return again.

A case history will show what the disease is like. At age seventeen, Nancy had a constant dull pain in her belly and a continual urge to move her bowels. A doctor gave her pills for the pain, but for years she was bothered by diarrhea and occasional constipation. At age thirty-two, she suddenly started painfully moving her bowels four times a day. Her diarrhea was accompanied by a frightening amount of blood and mucus. She lost weight, and was so pale and weak that she could not work. Finally, she went to a doctor and learned that she had ulcerative colitis.

A small number of patients with this disease develop complications similar to those found in ileitis: liver and kidney disorders, arthritis, skin lesions, and inflammation of the eyes. Colitis, like Crohn's disease, causes arrested growth and sexual development in children.

Ulcerative colitis is also a disease primarily of young people. Three out of four cases develop before age forty, and the victim typically is from an urban area in the industrialized northern United States, from the upper middle-class economic level, and is above average in intelligence and formal education. There is some evidence that ulcerative colitis may run in families. Apparently, it is twice as common among Jews as other groups. The National Foundation for Ileitis and Colitis estimates that ulcerative colitis and ileitis of varying severity may afflict two million Americans in all. About one hundred thousand new cases are diagnosed each year and, according to the NFIC, the incidence of these diseases appears to be on the rise.

The cause of ulcerative colitis remains a mystery. It may

be an infection, a sensitivity to certain foods, or a defect in the body's natural defenses, or "immune" mechanisms, that causes it to attack its own tissues. Environmental factors are also suspected, but the greatest controversy concerns whether emotional and psychological problems play a role. As Chapter 3 noted, the NFIC discounts any emotional causes of ileitis and ulcerative colitis. Yet some of the foremost textbooks on gastroenterology maintain that emotional conflict *does* play a major role in causing many, if not most, cases of ulcerative colitis.

A number of studies have shown that people with ulcerative colitis have trouble expressing — or even feeling — anger. They avoid confrontations and brood for weeks or months when their feelings are hurt. They are often dependent, tense, anxious, sensitive, depressed, and demanding. One study showed that threatened interruptions of key relationships tended to cause flare-ups of ulcerative colitis. These disruptions included family tensions, usually involving the mother; death or illness in the family; business tensions; and the stresses of romance, marriage, divorce, and discontent with the armed services.

Many people who have ulcerative colitis contend that their disease stems from physical, not emotional, causes. They say that colitis can cause considerable stress and subsequent emotional reactions of depression and anxiety, but that these are a consequence, not a cause, of their illness. They feel that if their colitis has emotional roots, it means they have caused their own illness, and are at fault for not being able to control their emotions.

Perhaps the greatest stress for ulcerative colitis and ileitis patients is the practical humiliation of experiencing acute pain in public, of carrying extra underpants and toilet paper in their purses and briefcases, and of always having to know where the nearest restroom is located, whether in a restaurant, department store, or subway station. Most stressful of all, they must learn to live with the reality that colitis, once established, will come back.

The drugs used to treat ulcerative colitis are palliative, that is, they relieve symptoms, but not causes. Drugs that relieve other forms of diarrhea will probably not relieve diarrhea caused by ulcerative colitis or, as noted earlier, ileitis. Sulfa-containing drugs such as Azulfidine and / or corticosteroid drugs are usually prescribed. The latter may be administered orally, by enema, suppositories, or injection. Corticosteroids are helpful, but long-term use of these drugs may cause a number of side effects, as mentioned in the earlier section on Crohn's disease. The treatment of ulcerative colitis largely depends upon the doctor's skill and the patient's cooperation. Psychotherapy sometimes helps people with ulcerative colitis deal with the stresses of the disease itself, their attitudes toward themselves and others, and with the underlying emotional factors that may have contributed to it.

During an attack of ulcerative colitis, you need bed rest and a high-protein diet to replenish nutrients. Some doctors prescribe a high-fiber diet to help control diarrhea. You also need to replace fluids lost through diarrhea. Sometimes abdominal cramps can be relieved at home with an electric heating pad or hot-water bottle, or by lying down after meals. Lying down also helps reduce the number of bowel movements.

If the attack is severe — involving high fever, significant bleeding, abdominal distention, drowsiness, or severe pain — you may have toxic megacolon, a serious complication of ulcerative colitis in which the colon dilates to four inches or more and acquires the consistency of wet toilet paper. Toxic megacolon is an emergency requiring immediate hospital care, intravenous feeding, and antibiotics. If the condition does not respond to this treatment within a day or two, and there is a strong possibility that the colon will perforate or bleed massively, the entire colon and rectum must be removed surgically.

Fortunately, only about fifteen percent of ulcerative colitis patients ever need surgery. The large bowel is not essential to life, and when it is removed by a procedure called a total colectomy, ulcerative colitis can be considered cured. Following this procedure, a surgeon draws the end of the small intestine through a hole in the abdominal wall, and attaches it so it protrudes slightly through the skin of the abdomen. This ileostomy, or "ostomy" as it is known, essentially is an artificial anus. It is then fitted with a bag which collects body wastes. A new type of "bagless" ileostomy is currently under development. The opening to the skin acts as a valve through which a tube must be passed in order to collect the stool. Not everybody is a candidate for this operation and, currently, very few surgeons are skilled in performing it. A surgical solution to ulcerative colitis — however difficult to live with — is sometimes far better than the disease. Surgical removal of the large bowel also eliminates the possibility of cancer of the colon and rectum — a risk that rises rapidly after you have had ulcerative colitis for ten years. Generally, people with ulcerative colitis should have a doctor check their colons for signs of cancer twice a year.

For years, research scientists have searched for a virus, bacteria, or autoimmune mechanism that causes ulcerative colitis, but no major discoveries are expected soon. There are studies of how this disease affects the body and its processes, and of how to make ulcerative colitis patients more comfortable. Scientists are also investigating the possibility that prostaglandins — hormonelike substances, found in almost every human cell, that regulate a wide variety of body activities — may prevent the development of colitis. In a study of hamsters, certain prostaglandins have been found to protect the mucous lining of the large intestine from inflammation. It is hoped that the same will prove true for humans. Earlier animal studies have shown that certain prostaglandins protect the lining of the stomach and small intestine from various noxious agents, including pure alcohol, strong acids, and aspirin. This new study of hamsters suggests that prostaglandins may protect the entire gastrointestinal tract.

While research continues on behalf of people with ulcerative colitis, most patients can control their disease and live reasonably normal lives. The disease often becomes inactive for long periods of time, and has even been known to "burn itself out." Even if ulcerative colitis becomes active and requires surgery, people who have had an ostomy can eat, drink, sleep, work, achieve career goals, make love, get married, give birth, and raise families. The United Ostomy

Association (see Appendix A) has forty-three thousand members and over 550 chapters throughout the United States. The Association helps the 1.5 million men and women in the United States and Canada who have had parts of their colons or urinary tracts removed, and who must eliminate body wastes through a stoma, or opening in their abdomens, into a bag. This support group, many of whose members have themselves had ostomies, helps "ostomates," as they are known, make the initial adjustments to colostomies, ileostomies, or urostomies.

The Association helps ostomates deal with such perplexing questions as: Will I smell? Will I bulge? Will I make noises? Will I feel waste leaving my body? Will I starve? Will I be a captive of the toilet? Will I be able to take baths, go swimming, bend over? Will I be a social outcast? Will I be able to get / stay married and have babies? The United Ostomy Association assures ostomates that they can swim, play football, sprint, box, climb mountains, and become test pilots and deep-sea divers. The Association also encourages ostomates to tell others about their surgery and about their ability to live full lives, even though parts of their intestines are missing. Such disclosure has promoted better public understanding, and has transformed negative attitudes about this once-dreaded operation into expressions of acceptance like, "You've sure got a lotta *guts!*"

Irritable Bowel Syndrome

Also known as spastic colon, irritable colon, unstable colon, mucous colitis, spastic colitis, nervous diarrhea or functional bowel disease, this is the "common cold" of the gastrointestinal tract. It does not kill you. It does not lead to cancer. But it does cause at least fifty percent of all digestive troubles! Irritable bowel syndrome is the one digestive disease doctors have long believed is emotionally induced. It has been called the "intestinal equivalent of weeping."

Irritable bowel syndrome is a functional disorder, that is, an abnormality in the behavior or function of the large bowel for which no organic cause has yet been found. When the functions of the colon are disrupted, the result is diarrhea and / or constipation with cramping abdominal pain, or painless diarrhea.

Your colon, like your stomach, receives nerve signals directly from your brain, by way of the hypothalamus. Few parts of your body are more vulnerable to psychological disturbances than your large bowel. When you are upset, you can feel your intestinal muscles tighten and contract. If you feel angry, resentful, anxious, or frustrated, your hypothalamus sends signals ordering your colon to "Wake up and get moving," and you might have diarrhea. If you feel dejected, it will tell your colon, "Hang on there," and you might be constipated. And yet, although you feel miserable, your bowel is not damaged or diseased. It is just out-of-kilter.

Many people who feel trapped by demands they believe they cannot meet are afflicted with irritable bowel syndrome. One study showed that patients with spastic colon had undergone more stress in the previous six months than unhospitalized subjects in the general population, and more than other patients in the study who had ulcerative colitis. Many of the spastic colon patients answered yes to these questions designed to measure life stress:

- Did either of your parents die before you were age sixteen?
- Was your father frequently unemployed?
- Have you been frequently unemployed?
- Do you and your spouse have different levels of education?
- Are you and your spouse of different religions?
- Have you been married more than once?
- Have you held three or more different jobs?
- Have you lived at three or more different addresses?
- Have you lived alone five years or longer?

The study also showed that many other precipitating factors or "triggers" had occurred during the six months before illness. These included physical injury, increased pressures at work, severe financial problems, loss of a job, serious family crises, and the death of a close friend or relative. The epidemiologists who conducted this study concluded that chronic illness may well occur in a setting of recurring despondency, in which the patient feels a significant loss or threat of loss, and feels helpless to do anything about it.

A later study of patients with spastic colon and ulcerative colitis described people in both groups as anxious, helpless, and unable to express their feelings. The self-avowed "nice guy," for example, or the good kid who never argues with his or her parents, or the sweet-tempered young wife might, deep down, be seething with anger, and yet be completely unaware of it. Such people are often amazed at how — once they learn to express their anger directly — their rampaging guts quiet down. Spastic colon patients have also been described as achievement-minded, intelligent, meticulous, sensitive, introspective individuals. It has been said that a spastic colon shows that the sufferer is striving for a better life. In that sense, the disease is a badge of distinction.

Irritable bowel syndrome commonly begins during adolescence and early adulthood and worsens during exams, marital or job troubles, financial stress, bereavement, the week before a menstrual period beings, and menopause. Irritable bowel syndrome is considered a disease of modern civilization. It is rare in the few remaining primitive cultures of the world, and is less common in rural than in urban areas. There is also some evidence that the disease runs in families.

A great many other conditions, including diabetes, vitamin deficiencies, food allergies, food poisoning, infections, parasites, acute illness, environmental factors, and metabolic disorders can cause the same symptoms as irritable bowel syndrome. In addition, many foods and agents can irritate the colon, including coffee, alcohol, spices, and fried foods.

Irritable bowel syndrome is somewhat of a wastebasket diagnosis for a number of annoying symptoms, including alternating attacks of diarrhea and constipation, and possibly gas pains or cramps on the left side. As a victim of the disease, you might also lose your appetite, belch frequently, and experience heart palpitations, shortness of breath, and fatigue after mild exertion. These symptoms occur because the heart and lungs are stimulated by the same parts of the nervous system as the colon. The symptoms are severe enough to send you to a doctor, who orders tests and finds they are all normal. You cannot understand how the tests can show nothing when you feel so bad. Stop and think: are you under any kind of stress? If the answer is yes, you may already start to feel better just from the reassurance of knowing the cause of your problem.

No one treatment works for irritable bowel syndrome, but many measures help:

- Avoid fried and other foods and spices that seem to make diarrhea worse.
- Avoid coffee, alcohol, and smoking.
- Eat slowly and chew food thoroughly, even to the point of fletcherizing.
- Drink plenty of fluids.
- Remember that fatigue or other illnesses, such as the flu, can cause irritable bowel disease to flare up.
- If you must, take Lomotil or belladonna to relieve occasional cramps and diarrhea, but do not take these drugs regularly.
- Do not resort to laxatives for constipation. Remember, they irritate the colon and can lead to laxative abuse (see Chapter 6).
- Increase the fiber in your diet by eating whole bran, fruits, and vegetables, or try bulk laxatives to relieve alternating diarrhea and constipation. Experiment to learn what dose produces regular bowel movements.

In theory, a high-fiber diet stabilizes the water content of the stool, preventing both constipation and diarrhea. Fiber also increases the volume of the stool and this, in turn, may stretch out areas of the colon in spasm, the same way you stretch out your leg to relieve a charley horse. The American Digestive Disease Society has developed a dietary plan to help people with irritable bowel syndrome (see Appendix A).

There is no surgical treatment for spastic colon. Some doctors prescribe mild sedatives, smooth muscle relaxants, and antispasmodic drugs for more severe cases. Scientists at The Johns Hopkins and Baltimore City hospitals are using biofeedback to teach patients to control the spasms of irritable bowel syndrome. They insert balloons into different sections of colon and inflate them to cause an abnormal spastic response. The patient, who sees the internal spasm recorded by means of instruments on a piece of paper, is told to try to suppress the spasms he sees on the paper. Two-thirds of the patients have been able to do so. Despite such promising studies, irritable bowel syndrome receives relatively little research attention, perhaps because it is not a killer disease.

The best remedy for spastic colon is to stop worrying about it or you will make it worse, and to avoid the stressful situations that produce the problem. It is not always easy to recognize the factors that cause stress and anxiety, nor is it easy to make effective stress-reducing adjustments in your work, family relations, and lifestyle. Dietary measures are helpful in this respect because diet is one factor you *can* control, and this sense of mastery can relieve many anxieties. You might also consider seeking help from a professional trained to deal with such problems, including a psychiatrist, clinical psychologist, family counselor, social worker, or clergyman. You can take solace in the likelihood that, as you become better equipped to handle life's problems, large and small, your spastic colon will gradually get better.

Appendicitis

Picture your large intestine as an upside-down U. Your appendix — if you still have one — dangles from the end of your large intestine on your right side, like an empty finger of a rubber glove. Hence, its name, the vermiform (wormlike) appendix. Rabbits, guinea pigs, and rats use their appendixes to digest grass, hard seeds, and bulk foods. The appendix is the largest part of their intestines, full partner in the digestive process. But the human appendix, a vestigial organ rendered useless by evolution, just hangs there, the bane of children aged six to twelve, and of many adults as well. It is one of the least understood and most frequently diseased organs in the body.

Suppose a vagrant speck of undigested food is pushed

into the neck of your appendix by the action of the intestines as they contract / relax / contract / relax. Somewhere along the appendix's four-inch length and $^3/_{10}$-inch diameter, the "fecalith" gets stuck. Or the unwelcome visitor may be of quite a different sort. Appendixes have served as a lodging place for nails, tacks, screws, and the seeds of fruits and vegetables. One surgeon found a germinating lima bean growing inside a newly removed appendix. As fecal and foreign matter packs against the lining of the obstructed appendix, the pressure stops blood from circulating, causing the already-irritated tissues to become swollen and inflamed. Once-friendly colon bacteria attack the dying tissues; gangrene sets in.

Appendicitis! The symptoms of inflammation of the appendix are familiar: sudden, sharp pain around the navel. It grows worse and, in a few hours, shifts to the lower right side of your abdomen or, if your appendix is not where it's supposed to be, perhaps to the left side of your abdomen. The pain may be continuous, dull or severe, and it may intensify if you press on your lower right side or move your right leg. You may become nauseated or vomit; your fever may climb to 102°F. A child's fever may soar even higher.

But the symptoms are not always so predictable. A young child may experience nothing more than vomiting, fever, and irritability, while some adults simply have persistent abdominal pain. If the pain lasts longer than three to four hours, you should call a doctor, for you may be in danger. Nor is appendicitis always simple to diagnose: gallbladder disease, kidney infection, pancreatitis, pelvic inflammatory disease in women, and even spastic colon produce similar symptoms, and must be ruled out before appendicitis can be diagnosed. This is one problem you should not self-treat. Home remedies like heating pads, cathartics, and enemas can only make matters worse since they obscure symptoms, intensify intestinal contractions and pressure, and may even cause the appendix to rupture.

A ruptured appendix will spill bacteria, pus, and stool throughout your sterile abdominal cavity and cause peritonitis. This could kill you unless a surgeon hastens to remove the diseased appendix, drain the abdominal cavity, and bring the infection under control with antibiotics.

Although appendectomy is the most common abdominal emergency in the United States — where about 260,000 of these procedures are performed annually — fewer than a thousand people die each year of appendicitis, nearly all of whom have peritonitis. A routine appendectomy is no longer considered major surgery. A small incision two to five inches long in the lower right side of the abdomen suffices. An appendix can be removed in as little as ten minutes, assuming there are no complications. You can go home from the hospital in five or six days, your incision completely heals in seven to ten days, and your appendicitis is cured forever.

As surgical procedures go, appendectomy is a relatively simple one that apprentice surgeons perform to gain experience. Men have been known to remove their own appendixes when there was no one else around to do it. "Autoappendectomies," however, are rare.

Why is the appendix so troublesome? Dr. Denis P. Burkitt, the British epidemiologist, argues that appendicitis is a disease of modern civilization. First described in England in 1812, appendicitis appears to have become common after 1880, when indigestible fiber began to disappear from bread and other carbohydrate foods. Appendicitis was rare among Africans before they replaced much of their traditional high-fiber diet with white bread, sugar, fat, and meat. The theory is that low-fiber diets lead to hard, small stools that do not fill out the colon and are too dry to pass easily. This causes the colon's muscles to overstrain and exert high pressure in order to push the stubborn mass along. The increased pressure caused by constipation and straining at stool are thought to damage the lining of the appendix, placing appendicitis on Burkitt's theoretical list of "pressure diseases," along with constipation, hiatal hernia, diverticular disease, hemorrhoids, and cancer of the colon.

It has also been suggested that appendicitis is a gut reaction to stress. Dr. Hans Selye, who for years has studied the relationship between stress and disease, notes that appendicitislike changes take place in certain animals exposed to very alarming stimuli. For example, during such conditions, the cecum of the rat, which corresponds to the human appendix, shows marked changes similar to those that occur during the first stages of acute appendicitis in man. The same reactions, Selye suggests, can take place in the human appendix, which contains a great deal of lymphatic tissue. Lymphatic organs, in turn, are known to be sensitive to adrenal hormones, which are released during prolonged stress. These hormones cause lymphocytes — or infection-fighting white blood cells produced by lymphatic tissues — to disintegrate. A final theory about why the appendix is so troublesome is that the intestines have not adapted anatomically to the human upright position.

Diverticular Disease

To develop diverticular disease, you must first have diverticula, or little pouches protruding outward from the mucous membrane that lines the intestine. This condition is called diverticulosis, from the Latin *divertere*, meaning to turn aside. The pouches range in size from a pinhead to a large grape. Most often they form, sometimes by the hundreds, in the weakest areas of the bowel wall, where small blood vessels enter the colon. Most diverticula form in the sigmoid section, or the last few feet, of the colon.

Diverticulosis, or the presence of many such pouches, is not a true disease. Most people who have diverticulosis do not even know it. Symptoms, if they develop, include gas, stomach cramps, and diarrhea alternating with constipation. Diverticulosis is rare in people under age thirty-five, and increases with age. One-third of Americans over age forty-five and two-thirds of those over age sixty have diverticulosis. Women are affected more often than men.

Diverticulosis may be caused by muscle shrinkage in an aging colon wall, or by an abnormal thickening of the wall. Many doctors believe that repeated blasting of the colon with powerful laxatives, purgatives, and enemas contributes to diverticulosis. Diverticula are also believed by some people to be the end products, as it were, of a lifetime of intestinal disturbances such as excess gas and chronic constipation.

Suppression of intestinal gas may cause diverticulosis because the descending gas is forced to return to the upper rectum and sigmoid, causing considerable pressure. Contributing to the gas theory is the fact that diverticular disease is confined to modern urban communities, where manners and morals require that gas — and often stools —be retained at any cost, whereas their retention in rural primitive societies is considered pointless.

Another support for this theory is the observation that the pain of diverticular disease, which usually occurs on the lower left side of the abdomen, is most noticeable in the evening, when gut activity and gas retention are at their greatest as the family gathers for the evening meal. And, if the previous points are unconvincing, it has been further noted that diverticular disease seldom occurs before ages ten to fifteen, which might be considered the dawn of social consciousness.

But the prime suspect for causing diverticular disease is the low-fiber diet so many Americans consume. Africans, Indians, Middle Easterners, and Orientals, who eat plenty of natural vegetable fiber, rarely develop diverticulosis, although in the upper socioeconomic groups in India and Iran the disease is beginning to make its debut. Diverticular disease wasn't even mentioned in medical textbooks until 1920, after which highly processed foods became popular.

According to Drs. Denis P. Burkitt and Neil S. Painter, the oft-cited British epidemiologists, the incidence of diverticular disease diminished in Great Britain during World War II. During this period, the amount of bran remaining in flour increased, white bread was not available, and refined sugar was strictly rationed. The same conclusion has been suggested by a clinical trial in which eighty percent of seventy diverticulosis patients who were fed a high-residue diet experienced relief of abdominal pain and distention. Yet, for years before the findings of Burkitt and Painter, a low-residue diet had been the mainstay of medical treatment for people with diverticular disease.

High-fiber foods, including bran (the outer coating of the whole wheat grain that is removed when grain is processed), cereals, celery, lettuce, and vegetables tend — once digested — to form into a soft, bulky mass that moves smoothly through the intestinal tract, and keeps the colon from narrowing. Such a wide-bore colon, Painter and Burkitt maintain, is less prone to diverticulosis. In addition, bulky stools, as noted in Chapter 1, pass through the intestinal tract in two days rather than four or five, and produce less pressure on that organ. Over time, small, hard stools produce unnatural stresses that cause sacs in the weakest areas of the colon's wall. For this reason, diverticulosis has been called a "pressure disease."

Painter and Burkitt also maintain that diverticulosis is a deficiency disease that, like scurvy (vitamin C deficiency), is completely preventable. Today, diverticulosis is second only to constipation as an affliction of the colon. Fiber deficiency is also a prime cause of constipation, which, in turn, contributes to — and probably causes — diverticulosis.

Most people can control diverticulosis *and* constipation by avoiding laxatives and cathartics, by farting freely, and by eating high-fiber foods. While diverticulosis can be controlled, once established, it will never go away.

About fifteen percent of people with diverticulosis develop diverticul*itis*, an infection of one or more of the sacs in the colon wall. These sacs trap fecal material, and may even perforate and bleed. Symptoms of diverticulitis include a steady, severe pain in your left side that will hurt more if you press down on that area. The pain is so like the pain that occurs on your right side during appendicitis that diverticulitis is sometimes called "left-handed appendicitis." However, just to show that nothing in medicine is simple, the pain of diverticulitis sometimes occurs on the right side as well. It may last minutes or days, and may be accompanied by fever, chills, gas pains, constipation, or alternating diarrhea and constipation.

If diverticulitis develops, you will be treated with bed rest, heat over your left side, a low-residue diet consisting of clear fluids to rest your bowel, stool softeners, and antibiotics to clear the inflammation. After the symptoms subside, you will go on a very soft diet and, after six weeks, your physician will probably gradually transfer you to a high-fiber diet. This can often control the problem and prevent the need for surgery. If the fever and severe pain persist, however, your doctor may recommend hospitalization. Diverticulitis is one of the leading causes of hospitalization in the United States.

Only about one in ten patients with diverticulitis needs surgery, usually for obstruction caused when the diverticula become abscessed. Or an inflamed pouch may burst and spill fecal matter into the abdominal cavity. Your physician may also recommend surgery if he suspects the possibility of cancer. According to epidemiological studies, diverticular disease, tumors of the large bowel, and ulcerative colitis are closely associated.

Surgery usually involves cutting out the diseased sections of the large bowel, and stitching the healthy sections together. If the bowel is extremely diseased, the operation may have to be done in stages, with an interval of several weeks between operations. Surgery for diverticulitis is no minor procedure — hospital stays of about ten days are required for each operation — but the chances for recovery are better than ninety-five in one hundred. The odds of never developing diverticulosis or *-itis* are extremely good, too — provided you eat a high-fiber diet and stop subjecting your colon to enemas and cathartics. Few digestive disorders are as easy to prevent — and treat.

Hemorrhoids

Back in the early 1960s, a surgeon from Springfield, Missouri, Dr. James T. Brown, wrote a little song to the tune of *Detour* that went:

> Now a man ain't no good,
> And he can't act like he should,
> If his seat of learning is so burning hot,
> If he's cautious when he walks,
> And a-frowning when he talks,
> Then you can bet here's what he's got:
>
> *Chorus:*
> Hemorrhoids —
> Always itching, always burn,
> Hemorrhoids

> Give you that look of concern,
> Hemorrhoids
> If you think your life is void,
> You should have
> A hemorrhoid.

Brown and five colleagues, known as "The Singing Doctors," also did songs about borborygmus, excessive gas, and appendectomies in which the surgeon couldn't find the appendix. The latter, sung to the tune of "On the Street Where You Live" from *My Fair Lady*, begins: ". . . all the nurses stared, They don't bother me, But the man behind my back was from Pathology . . ."

Hemorrhoids, which have moved some men to sing and others to swear, are one of mankind's oldest and most common afflictions. They have challenged physicians for four thousand years.

Up close, hemorrhoids — more colloquially known as "piles"— are no more than varicose veins in your anal canal that tend to stretch and enlarge with age. Hemorrhoids occur in two locations: in the mucous membrane lining of the rectum — in which case they are called internal — and / or in the muscular tissues of the anus — in which case they are called external.

Hemorrhoids may cause no problem at all. But when they enlarge, they may bleed from the rectum or visibly protrude through your anus, causing pain, itching, burning, and discharge. Four out of every five people who have hemorrhoids suffer some pain during a bowel movement, and some people with hemorrhoids also experience pain in the general rectal area. Perhaps recalling the surgical miseries of fifteen and twenty years ago, many hemorrhoid sufferers sit on their problem (sitting, in fact, helps produce it), rather than seek medical treatment. They suffer needlessly, and risk having undetected cancer as well.

To appreciate modern methods for removing hemorrhoids, you need only reflect upon the ancient medical arts in which hemorrhoids were pulled down with hooks, tied, cut, clamped, twisted, burned with hot irons, injected with creosote, and crushed. Consider this description of a treatment from the time of Hippocrates (460 B.C.):

Having laid him on his back, and placed a pillow below the breach, force out the anus as much as possible with the fingers, and make the irons red hot, and burn the pile until it is dried up, and so that no part may be left behind. And burn so as to have none of the hemorrhoids unburnt for you should burn them all up.

A little later, the great Roman medical historian Aulus Cornelius Celsus wrote in *De medicina:*

If a head (of a hemorrhoid) is very small and has a thin base, it must be tied with a flax thread a little above where it joins the anus. A large sponge squeezed out of hot water is next to be applied until it becomes livid; then with a finger nail or scalpel it is to be scarified above the knot. . . . If the head is larger and the base broader, it is to be seized by one or two hooks, and incision made a little above the base. . . . When the incisions have been made, a pin should be passed through, and under the pin the head is tied round with linen thread.

During the Middle Ages, quacks and barbers found willing hemorrhoid patients. A "surgeon" journeyed around the countryside, treating his victims in country inns while other customers looked on and his horse waited outside. A typical treatment of the day was described in 1269:

Thou shalt take a strong thread and knitte there aboute, and every dai thou schalte streine it more and more, till be falle awei and then with driying medicine thou schalt drie it up, or touche hem with an hoot iron that is bettere.

There were, to be sure, gentler treatments: ointments of acacia leaves, frankincense, myrrh, and celery. Moses Maimonides, the famed medieval physician, recommended in his *Treatise on Hemorrhoids* that the patient acquire a large earthen pot with a small hole in it, start a coal fire below the pot, and center his or her anus over the smoke hole three times an hour, once a week. And in Goethe's *Faust*, Mephistopheles tells of an apparent hemorrhoid sufferer who ". . . now will seat him in the nearest puddle, the solace this, whereof he's most assured . . ." (an early version of the sitz bath).

Hemorrhoids spared neither rich nor poor, famous nor obscure. Martin Luther suffered from piles and described them in long letters to friends. Cardinal de Richelieu, of the same era, counted hemorrhoids among his many afflictions, and had to use a litter to get around after riding a horse and walking became a torment.

During the Middle Ages, many of the afflicted prayed to St. Fiacre, healer of hemorrhoids and patron saint of proctology. This French holy man was somewhat of an all-purpose saint. Not only was he considered healer of all intestinal and anorectal miseries, he was also protector of gardeners and, as matters evolved, cab drivers (*fiacre* means "cab" in French). He was born around 600 A.D., first-born son of the King of Scotland. But because he preferred religion to politics, St. Fiacre refused to accept the throne of Scotland, and chose a hermit's life instead. At one point, he asked his bishop for some land, and was promised all the real estate he could surround with a ditch dug in one day. He dug a very long ditch, legend has it, and with only one stick. On his land he grew a beautiful garden full of vegetables and flowers, which provoked the envy of his neighbors, who accused him of witchcraft. To test his innocence, the bishop ordered St. Fiacre to sit for several days on a large stone at the church's door. But while he sat upon the stone, it softened and took on the imprint of the holy man's posterior, hence his reputation for curing hemorrhoids. (You need only sit on them, as St. Fiacre did on his stone, and keep faith.)

After St. Fiacre died quietly in 670 A.D., the stone became known far and wide for its miraculous healing powers, not only of hemorrhoids and anal bleeding, but of all anorectal disorders, and eventually of all intestinal ailments as well. As the remains of St. Fiacre's body were sawed up and sold for relics, his fame spread throughout Europe, and he came to be worshipped by gardeners as well. Historians consider it a paradox that today only a variety of bean bears his name. A recent issue of the *New Yorker*, however, carried an ad for a sculpture of St. Fiacre in his capacity as patron saint of gardeners. It stands twenty inches high, and is available for $250 from Florentine Craftsmen in New York City. And an ad that might have been inspired by St. Fiacre has appeared in New York City subways showing a woman cab driver saying, "I sit twelve hours a day. The last thing I need is hemorrhoids."

For centuries, it was believed that hemorrhoids were a reservoir into which the veins collected and later rejected waste. In the early eighteenth century, the Italian anatomist Giovanni Battista Morgagni observed that animals do not have hemorrhoids, and that perhaps their occurrence in man can be attributed to his erect posture. It was later theorized that hemorrhoids are caused by faulty blood circulation. In other words, blood was blocked because hemorrhoid veins supposedly had no valves to let it out. The idea that inflammation of hemorrhoidal veins causes the problem came along in the nineteenth century.

Today, hemorrhoids are thought to be weakened veins that, after stretching during defecation, fail to return to a normal state and remain permanently stretched. The swelling inside the rectum can become so pronounced that it obstructs the passage of stools. Under constant pressure, these weakened veins tend to rupture and bleed.

External hemorrhoids are often called "piles," from the Latin *pila,* meaning "ball," which is what many hemorrhoids look like. Some can even grow to the size of a golf ball, and many a hemorrhoid sufferer feels like he is sitting on one. These hemorrhoids around the anal sphincter contain many small nerves that make them painful and — when they become inflamed and infected — itchy as well.

Among the conditions known to cause hemorrhoids is pregnancy, particularly during the later months when the weight of the abdomen adds to the strain on the blood vessels of the anus. Such hemorrhoids usually disappear after childbirth. Hemorrhoids are also brought on by old age, sedentary living (they are an occupational hazard among airline pilots, for example), lack of exercise (which leads to constipation and poor blood circulation), insufficient fluid intake, prolonged standing, obesity, and overconcern with bowel function. But the foremost cause of hemorrhoids is thought to be excessive straining at stool, which causes pressures that dilate the veins in the rectum, and places hemorrhoids on the list of "pressure diseases." The straining, in turn, is caused by constipation. Conversely, hemorrhoids can lead to constipation if the pain they cause makes you delay or avoid going to the bathroom.

By some estimates, hemorrhoids afflict half of everybody over age fifty in this country, and one-fourth of people between ages twenty-five and fifty. Nor are children and teenagers immune. The scope of the hemorrhoid problem in the United States can be seen in sales of various remedies for this problem. The Food and Drug Administration estimates that Americans spend $80 million a year for over-the-counter hemorrhoid products, ranging from creams to suppositories and pile pipes (tubes for inserting ointments above the anal sphincter). Preparations containing zinc oxide may help soothe and toughen irritated tissue while your body heals the inflammation. But creams containing local anesthetics with names ending in "-caine" may, with repeated use, cause further irritation. No cream should ever be applied unless the area has been carefully cleaned — otherwise, you will trap bacteria beneath. In general, hemorrhoid preparations are of debatable value, and should never become a substitute for proper medical care, or a way of avoiding the embarrassment of admitting that you have piles.

In 1980, the Food and Drug Administration (FDA) issued a report on the ingredients in nonprescription drug products used for hemorrhoids, and noted that these ointments and suppositories are primarily for relief of *symptoms*, and not for the treatment of hemorrhoids. The FDA report said claims that state that certain products are safer or more effective than others are inappropriate and misleading. In other words, beware of hemorrhoid remedies claiming to be "medicinal," "doctor-tested," "nonnarcotic," and to contain "no stinging, smarting astringents." The FDA report also warned that over-the-counter anorectal drug products should not be used for children under twelve years old.

Home remedies for hemorrhoids include applying zinc oxide paste or powder to external hemorrhoids and relieving both kinds of hemorrhoids with hot baths, aspirin, stool softeners such as Metamucil, bed rest in a prone position, and an ice bag on your anus to relieve pain. Keep the anal area free of fecal matter with Tucks, or toilet paper moistened with water or your own saliva. It sometimes helps to apply direct finger pressure (with a clean finger) to push a prolapsed pile back into the rectum.

External hemorrhoids usually clear up in a few days and need no medical treatment unless home remedies fail to relieve them within a week. In general, hemorrhoids that cause no symptoms should be left alone. Skin tags, or enlarged areas of skin around the anus, are sometimes mistaken for hemorrhoids. They, too, should be left alone unless they cause inflammation or itching.

Even bleeding from hemorrhoids can be remedied at home unless it persists longer than a week. Blood from hemorrhoids is bright red and appears on the outside of the stool or on toilet paper. It is not medically significant unless it continues for several weeks. However, if you notice blood that is burgundy or black in color and is mixed into the stool, it is a sign of bleeding higher in the digestive tract, and is a serious matter that requires a doctor's immediate attention.

If hemorrhoids cause itching, burning, pain, and bleeding, or if they remain permanently protruded from your anus, see a doctor. Such symptoms, when they persist longer than a week, could signal a condition more serious than hemorrhoids, and should be treated in any event.

The real remedies for hemorrhoids must address the source of the problem. The best way to prevent them is to lose weight, exercise regularly, avoid prolonged standing and sitting, avoid excessive straining at stool, drink lots of fluids to prevent constipation, avoid laxatives, and eat a balanced diet containing fiber. Many a hemorrhoid sufferer has discovered that dietary measures alone have solved the problem.

Hemorrhoid treatment is of two types: medical or surgical, depending upon the severity of the problem and your wishes. Hemorrhoids may be treated in your doctor's office by injection with various chemicals to reduce their size. If a blood clot has formed in a hemorrhoid, your doctor may lance the vein and remove the clot.

Hemorrhoid surgery is seldom necessary and is needed only for the most persistent cases. For many years, it was essentially a refinement of the ancient tying and cutting methods, with the crucial addition of anesthesia. Old-style hemorrhoid surgery (even as recently as fifteen to twenty years ago) was extremely painful and often caused postoperative complications. Since then, techniques have vastly improved. The modern operation to remove hemorrhoids, called hemorrhoidectomy, is no longer considered major surgery. The procedure can be done without general anesthesia and usually takes less than half an hour. You may, however, experience considerable pain during the next three to five days, especially during bowel movements, and need about four days of hospitalization. Sitz baths — sitting in hot water — usually give relief, and within two weeks, the rectal area is again pain-free. Once removed by this method, hemorrhoids cannot recur, and for more than ninety percent of patients, other veins do not enlarge and turn into new hemorrhoids.

Since 1963, techniques for hemorrhoid removal have vastly improved. The method of rubber band ligation is used for internal hemorrhoids. Membranes over your hemorrhoid are tied with small rubber bands and pulled up so the hemorrhoid will no longer cause symptoms. The procedure is simple, relatively painless, and allows you to return to work the following day. In another version of this procedure, a doctor places a special latex band around the neck of the hemorrhoid. The band stops blood from circulating to the hemorrhoid, which dies and sloughs off in three to nine days. This may cause some itching, blood spotting, and a sensation of fullness, but the procedure causes little pain and can be done in your doctor's office.

Another procedure for treating hemorrhoids, which is popular in Great Britain, but not in the United States, is anal dilatation. The method was devised by a British physician, P.H. Lord, who believed that hemorrhoids are caused by constrictions or bands around the lower rectum and anal canal. His remedy was to give a patient general anesthesia, prop him up in an operating theater, and insert three or four fingers of *both* hands as far as they would reach into the lower rectum, dilating the passage in all directions. A plastic sponge measuring five by four by two inches was then inserted into the lower rectum and left in place for an hour. As soon as the patient recovered from the anesthesia — not to mention the rest of it — he was sent home and told to keep the back passage stretched by inserting a dilator for one minute each day for the next fourteen days, tapering off thereafter. The patient could return to work on the second day. Subsequent studies have questioned the nature of the abnormality this procedure corrects, but not its effectiveness.

An editorial in the *British Journal of Hospital Medicine* recently pondered the bewildering choice of procedures for treating hemorrhoids, noting that in days past,

. . . if big enough you cut them out, otherwise you injected carbolized oil. Then to disturb the peace of simple conviction came a Lord (1969) to show how forcible anal dilatation could do as well. . . . Thereafter the gates were wide open and the cosy assumptions of half a century irredeemably shattered.

If the old world has gone, though, who knows what to do in the new? 'To tie, to stab, to stretch, perchance to freeze' taunted the *Lancet* (1975), the rotters.

The "freeze" method that the British medical journal *Lancet* referred to is cryosurgery, which involves the freezing and destroying of hemorrhoidal tissue with a probe. This procedure, first reported in 1969, is relatively painless because it destroys local nerve endings. It requires no hospitalization or anesthesia. Unfortunately, rubber band ligation and cryosurgery may not prevent your hemorrhoids from recurring, unlike conventional surgery, which may hospitalize you, but is more likely to give you a lasting cure.

CHAPTER 11

Cancer of the Digestive Tract

Colo-Rectal Cancer — the Good News

A WOMAN WHO lives in Vienna, Virginia had just watched an American Cancer Society film warning that 102,000 people will develop cancer of the colon and rectum this year, and 52,000 people will die from it. "Why," the woman wanted to know, "does the United States have so much colo-rectal cancer?"

The American Cancer Society (ACS) recently conducted a nationwide survey of all educational and economic levels that provided one answer: most men and women over age eighteen know little or nothing about colo-rectal cancer, and have never had an examination that could help detect it. Another study showed that most women reporting to the Walter Reed Army Medical Center in Washington, D.C. thought that colo-rectal cancer occurs only in men. (Actually, the risk is equal for both sexes.) Other studies showed that only about fourteen percent of physicians were routinely examining patients for colo-rectal cancer. These findings suggest that the toilet taboo — and its embargo on anything to do with the rectum and anus — may have some bearing on why the United States has so much colo-rectal cancer.

Meanwhile, the answer many epidemiologists give is

170

that cancer of the colon and rectum is more prevalent in the United States because its people consume so many highly processed, low-fiber foods. Epidemiologists such as Dr. Denis P. Burkitt have reached this conclusion because colo-rectal cancer, like so many other digestive diseases, is rare in parts of Africa and India as well as in Japan, yet is far more common among Japanese migrants to the United States who apparently have adopted a Western diet. Colo-rectal cancer likewise occurs with much higher frequency among black Americans than among Africans.

Dr. Burkitt has also pointed out that most colon tumors occur in the part of the bowel where feces tend to stagnate. Thus, small stools moving slowly through the intestine might both increase the concentration of carcinogens in the stool, and prolong their contact with the colon, whereas the fast transit of fibrous food wastes through the large bowel gives cancer-causing substances less time to do damage.

There are also growing indications that diets high in fat and red meat may increase the risk of colon cancer. Although evidence is far from conclusive at this point, epidemiological studies show that bowel cancer is rare in rural Africa, where diets are low in animal fat and protein contained in red meat. In the United States, where bowel cancer is a major killer, almost half of the average American's daily caloric intake consists of fat. When rats and mice were fed a comparably fatty diet, they developed two to three times more colon cancer than animals fed a low-fat diet. Another study showed that Seventh-Day Adventists who had eaten fat at some point in their lives were several times more likely to develop colon cancer than those who had remained strict vegetarians.

According to a related theory, bile acids are the culprits. The more fat you eat, the more bile your liver produces. These extra bile acids apparently linger in your colon, where they may indirectly lead to the production of carcinogens, or cancer-causing substances. In support of this hypothesis, some British bacteriologists compared the stools of a group of forty healthy Englishmen, who came from an area where cancer of the large bowel is prevalent, with the stools of forty-eight healthy Ugandans, who came from an area where bowel cancer is rare. Results showed that bile salts in the stools of the Englishmen were far more broken down chemically — and presumably more capable of promoting the action of other cancer-causing chemicals — than those in the stools of the Ugandans.

Further evidence comes from studies showing that the Finns, who eat a high-fat diet similar to that of Americans, suffer a similar rate of heart disease but a far lower rate of colo-rectal cancer. Scientists speculate that the difference may stem from the high-fiber diet Finns consume. Their stools, which are two to three times bulkier than the average American's, may dilute the bile acids and pass them out of the body before they can cause damage.

Such research suggests that you can probably protect yourself from colo-rectal cancer by eating fewer highly processed foods. There is far more conclusive evidence, however, that you can protect yourself against significant harm from colo-rectal cancer by detecting it early.

One-fourth of all cancers occur in the digestive system, and the colon and rectum combined are the most frequent sites of malignancy within the body. Only lung cancer affects more men; only breast cancer affects more women. Despite its greater prevalence, more patients survive colo-rectal cancer than the deadlier, but less common, cancers of the esophagus, stomach, liver, and pancreas. The survival rate is better for colo-rectal cancer because it can be cured if detected early enough. Yet, many tumors of the large bowel still go undetected. An American Cancer Society (ACS) spokesperson explains why: "This is a type of cancer we don't talk about. Even today, 'stool,' 'bowel movement,' and 'rectum' are words many people can scarcely say to their doctors."

The ACS made prevention of colo-rectal cancer a number one priority in 1981. "Don't be embarrassed to death," was the message. And the intended audience was people over age forty, since ninety percent of colo-rectal patients are in that category.

For this group, the ACS recommends an annual physical that includes a digital examination. Your physician, by inserting a gloved finger into your rectum, can detect any cancerous areas that may be just inside your anus. If you are over age fifty, you should also have a proctosigmoidoscopy, or "procto" exam, yearly. For many people, the worst thing about this test is that it makes you feel so undignified. You must crouch on an examination table with your head down and rear end up, while a physician inserts a lighted tube the thickness of a broom handle into the first twelve inches of your rectum and lower colon to examine the lining for tumors and other abnormalities. One white-haired patient asked a gastroenterologist who had him up-ended on an examining table to perform this procedure, "Son, does your mother know what you do for a living?"

The test takes only about five minutes — it will seem like fifteen — and causes little more than a feeling of fullness and cramping. Unfortunately, many people are needlessly afraid of protosigmoidoscopy, and avoid this life-saving examination. Digital and "procto" examinations combined can detect sixty percent of all colo-rectal cancers (digital exams alone detect only twelve to fifteen percent), since most tumors occur in the lower third of your colon. Cancers detected by these tests have a high rate of cure.

A slightly lower percentage of colon cancers can be detected by a far simpler test that the American Cancer Society recommends that you do at home once a year if you are over age fifty. Since most colon cancers cause abnormal bleeding, the Guaiac test, as it is called, is designed to detect hidden blood in your stool. For at least forty-eight hours, you simply go on a meat-free, high-fiber diet that includes plenty of lettuce, spinach, corn, peanuts, and popcorn, and stay on it until you have collected specimens from three consecutive stools. These specimens are placed on a paper slide that has been presoaked with chemicals that detect the presence of blood. If there is any abnormality in your colon, the roughage passing through is likely to make it bleed. You collect stool samples from the toilet bowl with a wooden applicator stick, and spread a very thin smear on window A of the first slide. You then place a smear from another portion of the stool on window B. After your next two bowel movements, you repeat these steps and return the slides to your doctor.

In the unlikely event that the test is positive — that is, if blood is present in your stool, indicating the possibility of cancer — you will be advised to see your doctor immediately for further tests. Ninety-five percent of these tests for occult or hidden blood are negative, that is, they show no signs of cancer. Even positive results do not always mean you have cancer. The test is so sensitive that it can even detect bleeding gums. You are not supposed to take it during your menstrual period, or if you have a bleeding hemorrhoid. To obtain a test kit, ask your doctor, or call your local health department or local chapter of the American Cancer Society. If none is listed in your telephone directory, write to the national office of the American Cancer Society (see Appendix A) for the name of the chapter nearest you.

Many physicians and clinics now use this test to screen patients for cancer. But the test is not one hundred percent accurate. It may detect blood in the stool that comes from meat in the diet, or from minor, nonmalignant bleeding sources. More seriously, since cancers do not bleed continually, the test may fail to detect a malignancy in the colon.

Some controversies have developed in the scientific world about the need for mass screening of the population for colo-rectal cancer by means of this test. A panel of experts who convened for a meeting sponsored by the National Cancer Institute in June 1978 recommended against mass screening because there is not enough evidence at present to show that screening by stool occult blood testing reduces mortality from colo-rectal cancer. The panel, however, did recommend further evaluations of colo-rectal cancer screening using the Guaiac test. The panel also recommended that health professionals use the test only for symptom-free people over age forty, and for people with additional risk factors. The high-risk group includes people who have had ulcerative colitis for ten years or longer, people with a family history of bowel cancer or any other form of cancer, and people who have polyps (small, cherrylike growths on the intestinal wall that tend to become cancerous if they are not removed). If you are among those with a high risk of developing colo-rectal cancer, you may need more extensive testing, and should be under a physician's care.

Everybody, regardless of risk status, should know the symptoms of colo-rectal cancer: a change in bowel habits, such as sudden diarrhea or constipation or both in alternation, bright red or black blood in the stool, an increase in intestinal gas or pressure in the rectum, and vague abdominal discomfort or pain. See a doctor if any of these symptoms persists longer than two weeks. They indicate that a tumor may be obstructing the colon. The closer the cancer is to the rectum, the more pronounced these symptoms of obstruction will become. People who have hemorrhoids often ignore bleeding because they assume they know what is causing it. They are taking a big chance because, although hemorrhoids do not lead to rectal cancer, a tumor can coexist with hemorrhoids and go undetected. You must take responsibility for examining your bowel movements if you expect to notice rectal bleeding when it first occurs. In this respect, you might imitate the cat, who always looks at its end product before burying it in the litter box.

If you do develop colo-rectal cancer, take solace in the knowledge that about seventy percent of patients who have surgery for *early* colo-rectal cancer live at least five years after diagnosis and treatment, and many live much longer. Depending upon the type of cancer and the stage of the disease, a surgeon will remove the part of the bowel containing the tumor, and nearby lymph nodes that may spread cancer to other parts of the body. Radiation therapy and chemotherapy may be combined with surgery. The former is a treatment which bombards the cancer with X rays, cobalt, or other sources of ionizing radiation to damage or destroy cancer cells, while causing minimal damage to surrounding healthy tissue. Chemotherapy entails treatment with anticancer drugs that interfere with the growth of cancer cells. Since chemotherapy also destroys healthy tissues, your doctor must maintain a delicate balance between killing cancer cells and destroying too many normal cells. Sometimes, a combination of radiation therapy and chemotherapy is used instead of surgery.

However, surgery remains the best treatment for cancer of the colon and rectum. If extensive surgery is necessary to remove the entire lower colon, rectum, and anus — known as an abdominoperineal (AP) resection — the surgeon will also perform a colostomy and attach the end of the remaining colon to the abdominal surface, leaving an opening, or stoma, so that body wastes can pass into a bag that is attached to the abdomen. The colostomy may be temporary, to allow the bowels to rest for a while, but even if it is permanent, it will not impair bowel function, or prevent you from living an otherwise normal life (see Chapter 10). A new type of health professional, the enterostomal therapist, can help people with the physical and psychological problems of coping with a colostomy. Another important source of support is the United Ostomy Association (see Appendix A).

A study of over 220 patients with advanced rectal cancer has shown that recurrence of the disease was significantly reduced when surgery was combined with postoperative radiation and chemotherapy. Patients treated with surgery alone had recurrence rates of fifty-two percent, compared with twenty-one percent recurrence in patients treated with surgery plus radiation and chemotherapy. When researchers made this discovery during the study, they interrupted it and assigned those patients who were getting only surgical treatment to receive postoperative drug and radiation therapy as well.

Meanwhile, research scientists have developed a new procedure for destroying tumors by heat that may be an alternative to removing large sections of the colon. Studies of this procedure, called electrofulguration, suggest that it is as successful as AP resection in prolonging life for five years or more, but causes fewer complications and is far safer. The operation is performed under spinal instead of general anesthesia and takes about an hour. Patients are able to walk and eat the next day, and hospitalization is brief. This new method is still being evaluated to determine whether it is as successful as colostomy in prolonging life for five years or more.

Unlike the relatively optimistic outlook for people with cancer of the colon and rectum, people with cancer of the esophagus, stomach, liver, and pancreas have less favorable survival rates. Cancer of the gallbladder is particularly deadly. Surgery, chemotherapy, and radiation are ineffective against this disease, and most patients live only a few months following diagnosis. Fortunately, gallbladder cancer is also extremely rare: about four thousand Americans die from it each year, compared with the more than fifty-three thousand who die of colo-rectal cancer. Even rarer is cancer of the small intestine: it kills fewer than eight hundred Americans annually.

Cancer of the Esophagus

Cancer of the esophagus — a deadly disease that kills more than seven thousand Americans annually — appears to be linked to heavy consumption of alcoholic beverages and, to a lesser degree, to heavy smoking. Its most common symptom is difficulty in swallowing, or a feeling that swallowed food is sticking somewhere along the breastbone. Meat may be the first food to cause this sticking sensation, whether food is actually sticking or not. You also may feel a burning pain whenever you swallow food, which may last for moments or weeks, and comes from the area behind your breastbone.

To diagnose your problem, your doctor will ask you to swallow barium sulfate so that he can watch its progress on a fluoroscope machine as it flows into your stomach. This test, supplemented by X rays of the outline of the esophagus, reveals many abnormalities. It may also be necessary to examine the area with an esophagoscope, a slender instrument that is passed through your mouth and throat into your esophagus. Through this device, a doctor can inspect the entire length of your esophagus, remove a small tissue sample for biopsy, and wash the area with a solution that is retrieved and later examined for cancer cells from tumors too small to detect. If the tests show that you have cancer, you will be treated by radiation and, possibly, by surgery. Cancers in the lower part of the esophagus are more accessible to surgery than those in the upper esophagus. Scientists are looking for anticancer drugs to treat esophageal tumors, but at present, radiation and surgery are the main methods of treatment.

Stomach Cancer

Stomach cancer has been in decline for the past one hundred years. Still, more than fourteen thousand Americans die of the disease each year — twice as many men as women, and nearly all of them above the age of sixty. It is one of the deadlier cancers: survival rates five years after surgery run about thirteen percent. However, when this kind of cancer is detected *before* it has spread beyond the stomach, the survival rate runs as high as forty percent. The key to survival is early detection, and that depends upon knowing whether you are in a high-risk group and recognizing early symptoms. The foremost risk factor for stomach cancer is gastric ulcer, not so much because it may lead to stomach cancer, but because it can mask a malignancy. Among those at risk are people who have polyps in their colons and rectums, those who have previously had part of their stomachs removed or reattached to the small bowel, and people who are over the age of fifty, or who have pernicious anemia or undiagnosed symptoms in their upper digestive tracts.

The symptoms of stomach cancer may at first resemble those of many other digestive illnesses. If you have persistent indigestion, bloating, and discomfort after eating, slight nausea, loss of appetite, heartburn, or mild pain over the pit of the stomach for longer than two weeks, see a doctor. Later on, symptoms may become more severe: vomiting, weight loss, pain, and red or black blood in the stool, which can be an indication of cancer anywhere in the intestinal tract, including the stomach. The problem is that by the time these symptoms occur, a malignant tumor may have been present for up to twenty months, and may have started to spread beyond the stomach to other organs.

If there is any suspicion of stomach cancer, your doctor will test your blood and stool, and order an X ray examination of your stomach. In some cases, you may need to see a specialist who will examine the inside of your stomach with a flexible lighted tube, which is passed through your mouth into your stomach. This instrument, called an endoscope, can detect a small growth and cut off a small piece of it for microscopic examination — a procedure known as biopsy. Although it is not pleasant to have an endoscope snaking around in your stomach, the test takes only about ten minutes and usually has no aftereffects.

Should test results show that you have stomach cancer, immediate surgery is essential. It may be necessary to remove most or all of your stomach, along with lymph nodes and adjoining tissues. If the entire stomach is removed, the surgeon will connect your esophagus to your duodenum, which will take over the digestion of food. You will have to eat small, frequent meals throughout the day, instead of the usual three large ones, and your diet will be low in carbohydrates and high in protein and fat.

Liver Cancer

Most of the fifty thousand people who are afflicted with liver cancer each year have the kind that has spread from another part of the body. This spread, or metastasis, from other organs occurs because of the liver's key position in the blood circulation system. Cancer may also originate in the liver, in which case it is called primary liver cancer. If liver cancer of either type is detected at an early stage, while the tumor is still well encapsulated and confined to one of the two lobes of the liver, it can be treated by surgically removing one of the lobes. But most cases of liver cancer are not detected in time and have a very poor prognosis.

A recently developed implantable infusion pump promises to prolong survival in cases of primary and metastic liver cancers that are not too advanced. The pump — which is being implanted surgically by Dr. William D. Ensminger and colleagues at the University of Michigan — delivers up to four hundred times the amount of powerful cancer-fighting drugs that the body can usually tolerate. The pump is still highly experimental, but, thus far, tumors have been significantly reduced in about eighty-five percent of the cases, and life expectancy has been extended from half a year to longer than two years.

Not much is known about cancer that originates in the liver, except that it appears to be associated with exposure to certain parasites, drugs, and to chemicals like polyvinyl chloride, and to heavy metals. It is not very common in the United States — only about twelve thousand cases of primary liver cancer are diagnosed annually — but it is widespread in many Asian and African countries, where most people have been exposed to the hepatitis B virus. Consistent with this observation, research scientists from the Institute for Cancer Research in Philadelphia recently reported that primary liver cancer seems to be preceded in nearly all cases by infection with the hepatitis B virus. People who carry this virus have a two-hundred-fold greater chance of developing primary liver cancer than people who do not harbor hepatitis B virus. However, this does not mean the virus is the sole cause of liver cancer; hepatitis B virus may merely set the stage for other substances that cause malignancy in that organ.

These findings suggest that it may become possible to diagnose liver cancer early by periodically giving cancer-detecting blood tests to known hepatitis B carriers. The research also suggests that the newly developed vaccine against hepatitis B virus may eventually become a way of preventing liver cancer. But the effectiveness of hepatitis B vaccine against liver cancer will not be known for many years because that disease apparently takes about thirty years to develop after the initial hepatitis infection.

Pancreatic Cancer

Cancer of the pancreas has evolved from a rare disease in the first half of this century to one of today's more common human cancers. The annual incidence of pancreatic cancer has tripled since 1930, and it is now the fourth most common cause of cancer deaths in the United States. About twenty-two thousand Americans die of it annually. Only cancers of the lung, colon, and breast kill more people. About three percent of people who were diagnosed as having pancreatic cancer between 1950 and 1973 survived for three years.

When cancer cells invade the pancreas, they most often affect its duct system. The earliest symptom is usually abdominal pain that radiates to the back. At first, the pain may come and go, but eventually it becomes persistent. If cancer develops in the head of the pancreas where the main pancreatic duct joins with the common bile duct, it may block that duct, causing bile back-up and jaundice. A rare form of pancreatic cancer affects the cells that produce and secrete insulin. This condition, islet cell cancer, may cause overproduction of insulin, which reduces the amount of sugar in the blood and leads to dizziness, chills, double vision, muscle spasms, and, sometimes, coma.

If the cancer is confined to the head of the pancreas, this part of the organ may be removed surgically, thereby curing the disease. Sometimes a malignancy is so large that it cannot be entirely removed even though it is blocking the bile duct. It may be possible to "short circuit" the bile duct by connecting the gallbladder to a loop of small bowel so that bile can bypass the obstructed duct. In an even more unusual surgical feat, it is now possible to remove the entire pancreas and compensate for its absence with diet and medication.

Pancreatic cancer is concentrated in Western industrial countries and in certain racial groups, including native Hawaiians and black Americans. It is very prevalent among people over seventy-five years old, among diabetics — who have a twofold greater risk of developing it — and among people who smoke cigarettes — whose risk is 2.5 times greater than the risk of nonsmokers. There also seems to be some relationship between incidence of pancreatic cancer and consumption of fat and cholesterol.

Recently, coffee use has been associated — statistically, at least — with cancer of the pancreas. Harvard epidemiologists interviewed 369 patients with pancreatic cancer and compared them to a "control" group of 644 patients with other cancerous and noncancerous diseases. The researchers found little or no association between cigarette smoking, tea, and alcohol consumption and cancer of the pancreas. But they did find, to their surprise, that people in the study who drank two cups of coffee a day ran twice the risk of developing pancreatic cancer as noncoffee drinkers. People who drank more than five cups a day ran more than three times the risk of nonusers. From this statistical association, the

Harvard epidemiologists suggested that more than half the pancreatic cancer in the United States might be attributable to coffee drinking. They urged that further studies explore whether coffee actually causes cancer of the pancreas.

These findings have provoked considerable controversy in both commercial and scientific circles. The National Coffee Association issued a statement noting that the Harvard study did not claim any cause-effect relationship between coffee and pancreatic cancer. Numerous scientists have criticized the Harvard investigators for their research methods and for comparing pancreatic cancer patients with patients hospitalized for noncancerous digestive diseases who may be underconsumers of coffee because of their health problems. Other critics noted that the study does not show whether the reported increase in pancreatic cancer reflects new cases or improved methods of identifying the disease.

Cancer Prospects — Better Than You Think

No disease provokes such widespread fear as cancer, and with the fear comes a terrible sense of helplessness. Most people equate cancer with death, disability, and disfigurement, and do not realize that great progress has been made against the disease, especially in the last ten to fifteen years. According to Dr. Vincent T. DeVita, Jr., director of the National Cancer Institute, half of all cancer patients in the United States could live the rest of their lives without a recurrence of their cancer if they took advantage of currently available diagnostic and treatment techniques such as proctoscopy or the Guaiac test, which allow early detection of colo-rectal cancers. Many cancer patients do not take advantage of the best treatments medicine has to offer. For example, many are reluctant to participate in clinical trials designed to discover which cancer treatments are the most effective. This reluctance to participate means it will take longer to discover improved ways of treating cancer. Nor are the human "guinea pigs" in these clinical trials at any medical disadvantage. Experience has shown that ninety-five percent of the patients receiving experimental treatments did better than patients who did not try the newer therapies.

A second factor that makes cancer more prevalent than it need be is that so many people do not avoid known causes of the disease. Cigarette smoking is a dramatic case in point. The intestinal tract is a prime target organ for cancer since it comes in contact with all the food and water you consume, plus a significant amount of the substances you inhale — twenty percent of which you actually swallow. Thus, the airborne environmental agents that you inhale directly expose your intestines to cancer-causing substances, known as carcinogens.

A third factor is that people do not adopt healthful practices that appear to prevent cancer. A high-fiber, low-fat diet, for example, is probably the best insurance against cancer of the colon, and many other digestive disorders.

Finally, many people do not know whether they are in a high-risk group for cancer of the colon or liver, or for some other serious digestive disorder. Whether you are in a high-risk group or not, you should learn the warning signs of cancer or other serious diseases of the digestive tract. They include:

- Severe, persistent (longer than six hours), or unexplained pain.
- Sudden changes in bowel habits.
- Blood in your stool or vomitus.
- Gray or clay-colored stools.
- Persistent or recurring fever of 101°F. or higher.
- Sudden loss of weight or appetite.
- Jaundice or dark urine.
- Difficulty swallowing food.

If any of these symptoms occur, see your doctor immediately. Cancer is a great masquerader and may imitate any number of other digestive diseases described in this book. Only your doctor can answer the question, "What is wrong with my gut?" But only *you* can ask it, and hopefully you will do so before cancer — or any other digestive ailment — gets out of control.

CHAPTER 12

Young Guts and Old

THE IMMATURE digestive tract is vastly different from that of the adult. From a germ-free environment, the newborn gut must adapt to a variety of bacteria. The symptoms of many digestive diseases are different among children than among adults. For example, at one time, peptic ulcer was considered very rare in children because the symptoms were difficult to detect. Today, ulcers are increasingly recognized as a disease that afflicts children. Certain chronic intestinal disorders hit hardest at adolescents and young adults, often subjecting them to a lifetime of drug therapy and surgery and, when they strike before puberty, retarding their growth and sexual development.

Colic

One of the first, and most common, digestive distresses of babies aged one to three months is colic, or painful spasms in the intestine caused by "gas" — actually, the peristaltic activity of the stomach. Colic appears to be triggered by tension and fatigue in an immature nervous system rather than primarily by diet. To manage this problem, keep yourself and your baby calm, lay the baby, stomach down, over your knees or over a hot water bottle wrapped in a towel. Many parents find that their child's distress is lessened by riding in a car, rocking, or swinging gently in a mechanical swing. Colic attacks may occur periodically during the first three months, or, in more severe cases, they may occur every night for three months or longer. If colic is severe, or if you feel unable to deal with it, talk to your pediatrician.

Infant Diarrhea

Diarrhea, in contrast to colic, is a very serious ailment of babies and young children because they have a very small water reserve, and diarrhea causes a significant loss of body fluids through the bowels. During the first two years of life, a baby's intestines must adapt to bacteria that don't bother older children and grownups. While an adult can tolerate diarrhea for two or three days before it is necessary to call a doctor, a baby may need a doctor's immediate care even for a mild case, because dehydration from this disease may quickly become a serious threat to an infant's life. Immediate treatment will lessen the severity of diarrhea and its consequences.

Your baby has diarrhea if bowel movements suddenly turn loose and become more numerous. It may be important to note if bowel movements change color (usually to greenish) or have a different odor. Infant diarrhea is an emergency and the child should be taken to a doctor or to a hospital immediately if:

- Stools suddenly become loose or watery.
- Stools contain pus or blood.
- Fever rises to 101°F. or more.
- Vomiting occurs.

When diarrhea strikes children aged two and older, keep your child in bed and administer fluids and soft foods. Scientists are trying to develop an effective vaccine to prevent acute viral infections of the digestive system that have such serious consequences early in life (see Chapter 7).

◇   ◇   ◇

Vomiting

Another cause of fluid loss in young children is vomiting, which also may be caused by stomach flu. Vomiting may also accompany a variety of other illnesses, including pneumonia, food poisoning, head injury, or intestinal obstruction. Dehydration — evidenced by extreme thirst, dryness of the mouth, listlessness, and "doughy" skin — is a threat if a child under two years loses all fluid from vomiting and diarrhea for six hours, or if a child between two and ten years old loses all fluid for eight to ten hours. The appearance of vomit is also important: if it appears black or bloody, it could mean internal bleeding; if it contains green bile, it could be a sign of intestinal obstruction. Such symptoms require immediate medical attention. If vomiting is less severe, give your child replacement fluids, such as water, flat ginger ale, bouillon, and soups. But you should administer these gradually — one-half ounce at first, working up to four ounces at a time the first day. If fluids cause the child to vomit again, he or she will probably lose more than you have just tried to replace.

As noted in Chapter 5, some children vomit because they feel tense and nervous, or have suffered some other emotional trauma such as the loss of a parent. Vomiting can also become a way of getting attention, or of avoiding something unpleasant, like school. Sometimes a child vomits on school days because he or she is not yet adapted to the new environment or to a new teacher.

Sometimes a child swallows something he should not, and emergency treatment cannot wait until you get him to the nearest hospital emergency room. First call your doctor or a Poison Information Center and ask what to do. If you cannot reach either source immediately, give your child syrup of ipecac, unless he or she shows signs of convulsions, severe pain, or burning in the mouth or throat. Read the list of substances on the label for which you should not induce vomiting. These include petroleum-based compounds like kerosene and gasoline, cleaning fluids, lighter fluid, toilet bowl cleaner, turpentine, ammonia, bleach, insect sprays, liquid furniture polish, and strong acids and alkalis. Then take your child to the nearest hospital or emergency room and carry the syrup of ipecac along in case the first dose does not cause vomiting in fifteen minutes. Your medicine cabinet, needless to say, should include a bottle of this emergency remedy if you have small children.

Constipation in Children

Constipation is another problem of babies and older children. Most babies have several bowel movements a day, and older children usually have at least one, but frequency can be an individual matter, just as it is among adults. Often children will become constipated when they are ill, especially with fever. Your child has a problem only if constipation is accompanied by painful bowel movements, excessive straining at stool, or long periods between bowel movements marked by malaise and a loss of appetite.

Children can become constipated for psychological reasons, just as adults do. The triggering events may be reaction to difficult toilet-training, or fear of having painfully hard bowel movements, after having had them at some point in the past. Such withholding may lead to even more serious constipation.

Try home remedies first. For babies, it often helps to add a teaspoon or two of corn syrup to their formula, or to give them prune juice or stewed prunes. For older children, the remedies are the same as for adults. Increase the amount of roughage in the diet, and make sure the child drinks plenty of fluids and gets adequate exercise. If these remedies fail, don't resort to laxatives, mineral oil, or enemas. Ask your doctor how to soften your child's stools.

Celiac Disease

Inability to digest certain foods can cause a variety of digestive problems in young children, including diarrhea that emerges as a foul-smelling froth containing undigested particles of food. Abdominal pain, gas, bloating, and stools that float are also common symptoms, and any child who has them should be taken to a doctor. These symptoms may be caused by celiac disease, a sensitivity to gluten — a protein found in wheat, barley, oats, buckwheat, and rye. This disorder, also known as celiac sprue, causes changes in the small intestine that make it unable to digest food, and thus, is called a malabsorption disease. If left untreated in small children, celiac disease can cause them to become weak, wasted, and undernourished, and may even stunt their growth. Fortunately, this disease can be treated, although complete recovery may take a year. All you need do is eliminate products containing wheat, oats, barley, buckwheat, and rye from your child's diet. You may substitute corn, rice, soy, potatoes, beans, and wheat starch from which the gluten has been removed. Celiac disease tends to run in families, and at least ten percent of those afflicted have other family members with the disease.

Lactose Intolerance

Another condition that affects people of all ages, but is often discovered in childhood, is lactose intolerance, or the inability of the small intestine to properly absorb the major sugar in cow's milk. Whenever the child drinks milk or eats milk products, undigested lactose reaches the colon, and bacteria change it into products that can cause bloating, excessive gas, and recurring abdominal pain. Thus, the child who refuses to drink milk may sense something you do not. Once the problem is identified, the solution is to avoid these foods.

Sometimes, however, identifying the problem is not easy. One woman suffered for years from gas and bloating, and had her gallbladder, uterus, and ovaries removed by doctors trying to cure her problem. Only when her problem persisted did doctors discover that the cause all along had been insufficient amounts of the enzyme (lactase) that digests milk.

About thirty million adults in the United States are mildly intolerant of lactose and experience symptoms only when they overindulge in milk, cheese, ice cream, or other milk products. Often they do not realize that they are lactose intolerant. One clue is that diarrhea caused by this condition usually occurs from thirty to sixty minutes after overeating such foods.

Thus, lactose intolerance does not always mean you must avoid milk entirely, just to the degree necessary to ease symptoms. For children who are intolerant of milk, milk substitutes can be used. But those who are completely intolerant of lactose must eliminate all dairy products from their diet, including nonfat or dried milk or cream, sour cream, butter, cheeses, yogurt, custards, and all products containing milk or milk solids and butter. This requires reading food labels carefully for hidden listings of nonfat dried milk and milk solids.

Lactose intolerance is extremely common among children in many parts of the world, including the Mediterranean and Asia. It is less common among Caucasians, whereas most blacks become lactose intolerant as adults. This casts some doubt on dairy industry claims that "you never outgrow your need for milk." One group of mammals born without a need for milk includes the seals, sea lions, and walruses of the Pacific basin. They have no lactose in their milk whatsoever, and get very sick if they are given any. This was not realized back in 1933, when a baby walrus being shipped from Alaska to California was fed cow's milk. The walrus suffered severe diarrhea throughout the voyage.

Sometimes children who cannot drink cow's milk are allergic to one or more of the proteins in milk. This, strictly speaking, is a food allergy. The baby may later be able to drink milk, but until that happens, the treatment is the same as for lactose intolerance: avoid it. The symptoms of milk allergy are far more varied than those of lactose intolerance, and may be difficult to recognize. They include colic, diarrhea, eczema (skin inflammation), constipation, asthma, ear infections, excessive fatigue, refusal to eat, and irritability. Milk allergy is more likely to occur if a child is fed cow's milk before the age of six months. The least likely cause of such an allergy is human breast milk.

◇   ◇   ◇

Abdominal Pain

Abdominal pain is a common childhood symptom, and is usually caused by stomach flu or constipation, rather than by something more serious. Emotional upsets can also cause abdominal pain in children, especially if no other symptoms accompany it. Sometimes it is difficult to determine whether the cause is physical or emotional, but if abdominal pain lasts longer than a few days, you should take your child to a doctor. *Very severe* abdominal pain that lasts longer than five hours may be more serious and should be referred to a doctor, especially if accompanied by appetite loss, vomiting, or fever.

It is possible that appendicitis is the cause of abdominal pain, although this disease seldom occurs in infancy. Often the only warnings in young children are vomiting, fever, and irritability. Sometimes there isn't even any fever or vomiting. The child may lose his or her appetite, but not necessarily. Even doctors have trouble diagnosing appendicitis in children. The strongest indication they usually find is tenderness when they examine the child's right side. Appendicitis is more common among teenagers and young adults, whose symptoms are more like those of an adult (see Chapter 10).

Childhood Ulcers

Ulcer symptoms in very young children differ from those in adults. A child's ulcer pain, if it occurs at all, tends to occur at night, when adult gastric secretions are greatly reduced. Young children with ulcers also become nauseated and vomit — a most unusual occurrence in adults — and the nausea may be worse on school days. This causes many a parent to misinterpret its origin. Another problem is that very young children have trouble describing their symptoms. Parents must watch for vague abdominal pain that lasts several days and then disappears for weeks or months, for blood in the stool or in vomitus, and for tendencies to eat poorly.

Doctors treat children's peptic ulcers with antacids, cimetidine, diet, and psychotherapy. Ulcer surgery for very young children is rare. Not until recent years were ulcers even recognized as a possible problem in children. In 1959, a Childhood Peptic Ulcer Registry was started to keep track of unpublished cases. Since that time, the number of cases reported has made it clear that peptic ulcer is no rarity, even in the newborn.

The reasons that children develop ulcers are not well understood, but one study of peptic ulcer disease in preadolescents and adolescents in New York showed that this disease may be associated with real or threatened loss of a loved one (a close family member or personal friend), by physical separation or divorce, or with potential loss from a life-threatening illness. Of twenty-three young ulcer patients studied over a ten-year period, it was found that ten had suffered such a loss during the twelve months preceding hospital admission, and five had suffered a significant loss within three weeks of admission to the hospital. The physicians who conducted the study concluded that such losses may affect the *timing* of an ulcer's occurrence in predisposed children and adolescents, and not the occurrence of ulcers per se.

Another study suggests that certain children and adolescents may be predisposed to ulcer disease. Research scientists have now shown that elevated concentrations of pepsinogen in the blood is inherited and is associated with duodenal ulcer. Other studies show that close relatives of persons with ulcers are three times more likely to develop ulcers than the general population.

Liver Disease in the Young

More than a hundred different liver diseases afflict infants and children. Tens of thousands of American children develop these diseases and many, especially babies, die from them annually. Frequently, diseases of the liver and bile ducts are caused by genetic or developmental abnormalities, or by damage to the liver that occurs during pregnancy or shortly after birth. These conditions can permanently damage the liver, brain, and other organs if they are severe and are not prevented by such therapies as exchange transfusions of the infant's blood, or by drug treatment of the mother during the last few days of pregnancy.

Hepatitis A is the most common childhood liver disease, and affects millions of children throughout the world (see Chapter 9). But once it runs its course, recovery is nearly always complete. The same cannot be said of hepatitis B or neonatal hepatitis, which can be transmitted from a pregnant woman to her baby. Children infected with this agent may develop chronic hepatitis, which gradually destroys normal liver cells, replaces them with scar tissue, and makes the liver unable to function properly.

One of the less common childhood liver diseases is biliary atresia, a condition in which the bile ducts leading from the liver to the small intestine are absent or too small to excrete bile. Although experimental surgical procedures continue to be developed, most severely affected infants die from cirrhosis by the age of two. Children may also develop liver disease due to galactosemia, an inherited absence of galactase, an enzyme needed to digest galactose, a milk sugar. This causes galactose to build up in the liver and other organs, leading to cirrhosis of the liver, cataracts, and brain damage. The cure is to take the child off milk.

Wilson's disease, which also afflicts children, causes large amounts of copper to build up in the liver and other tissues, leading to cirrhosis and brain damage. Reye's syndrome is another serious disease, in which the child goes into deep coma as the liver and other organs undergo a fatty degeneration. It is one of the ten leading causes of death in children beyond the age of infancy. You should suspect Reye's syndrome in a child who, while recovering from chicken pox or influenza, unexpectedly begins to vomit, and shows behavior changes such as lethargy, confusion, irritability, or aggressiveness.

Cirrhosis of the liver, the end result of most of these disorders, can be caused by any extensive injury to the liver. Such injuries can be caused by drugs, alcohol, infection, or by chemical exposure such as glue sniffing.

Alcoholic liver diseases are increasingly afflicting young adolescents who consume large amounts of alcohol. Even the unborn child can be harmed if the mother has been taking as few as two drinks a day. Indeed, the Surgeon General of the United States issued a warning in July 1981 saying that pregnant women should avoid *all* alcoholic beverages since problems — ranging from decreased weight at birth to malformations and birth defects — had occurred in infants of women who drank as little as *one ounce* of alcohol twice a week. The warning resembles one that appears in the Book of Judges (13:7): "Behold, thou shalt conceive and bear a son; and now drink no wine or strong drink . . ." (The son, born to the wife of Manoah, was Samson, whose great strength became legendary.)

Parents should seek genetic counseling if there is a family history of liver disease, and should learn the symptoms of disturbed liver function. The most obvious warning is jaundice, or yellowing of the skin and whites of the eyes. Other changes you should watch for include:

- Dark urine.
- Gray or light-colored stools.
- Nausea and vomiting of blood.
- Black or bloody stools.
- Loss of appetite.
- Abdominal swelling.
- Prolonged generalized itching.
- Unusual change in weight.
- Abdominal pain.
- Fatigue and loss of stamina.
- Sleep disturbances.
- Mental confusion or coma.

Bowel Disorders and Hemorrhoids

As mentioned in Chapter 10, children and young adults frequently are victims of ileitis and ulcerative colitis — two severe inflammatory bowel diseases. In about fifteen percent of the afflicted, these diseases first occur before the age of sixteen. Retarded growth or delayed onset of puberty may be the only symptoms in children, whereas adults suffer the dramatic bouts of abdominal cramps and bloody diarrhea.

Parents should be alert for youngsters who fail to grow or thrive and who feel sick and complain of weakness, for these symptoms could indicate that they have inflammatory bowel disease.

In rare instances, hemorrhoids occur in children under twelve years of age. When they do, they may have a serious cause such as obstruction of a major blood vessel or liver disease. A doctor should be consulted immediately, and over-the-counter hemorrhoid remedies should *not* be used. Small streaks of blood on the outside of bowel movements may be caused by a crack or "fissure" in the child's anus caused, in turn, by hard bowel movements. Light bleeding is no cause for alarm, but you should consult a doctor about treating the underlying constipation. It is a rare event when a child's stool contains large amounts of blood. This may indicate a malformation or other abnormality of the intestines, or severe diarrhea. Again, in such cases, call your doctor right away.

The Old Gray Gut

The gastrointestinal tract causes the elderly more trouble than any other body system. Yet, the digestive problems of old people do not differ greatly from those of the young, and problems that do occur cannot be attributed to "wear and tear" on the aging gut.

As you grow older, you are more likely to experience "irregularity," stomach pain, diarrhea, gas, nausea, and vomiting, all of which are usually caused — at any age — by factors you can control. For example, the foremost remediable complaint of the older person is constipation, and the main causes are lack of fiber in the diet and diminished physical activity. Other causes include inadequate fluid intake, poor eating habits, and habitual use of laxatives and cathartics. Among the psychological roots of constipation are anxiety and depression.

Constipation rarely indicates a more serious disease, and you seldom need a doctor or drugs to treat it unless it is particularly severe. Nor do you need laxatives, mineral oil, or enemas, although particularly resistant cases may need some stimulation from below. What you need, most of all, are fresh and cooked fruits, raw vegetables, whole grain cereals and breads, and bran in your diet, along with abundant liquids. And you need exercise, in the form of walking, swimming, bicycling, gardening, or some other physical activity.

Old people occasionally develop a fecal impaction that may require a doctor's finger or an enema to break it up. Fecal incontinence is another important complication of constipation in the elderly. If the constipation were treated properly, this problem could also be eliminated.

Many older people live in constant dread of cancer, even though it is much less likely to lie at the root of their symptoms than numerous other digestive ailments. Advances in diagnostic and surgical techniques have improved the outlook for treating gastrointestinal cancer. Even the dread cancers of the colon and rectum can be cured if detected early enough. If you are over age fifty, you should have a "procto" examination of your rectum and lower colon at regular intervals as recommended by your doctor, and you should self-administer the Guaiac test for hidden blood every year. (see Chapter 11).

The stomach is one organ that does seem to change with aging. These changes may cause a number of digestive problems in older people, including gastritis, or inflammation of the lining of the stomach, peptic ulcers, and inflammation of the esophagus. Any of these conditions may cause the steady, burning pain of heartburn at the tip of your breastbone (see Chapters 5 and 9). To treat heartburn, take nonabsorbable antacids like Maalox, Mylanta, or Gelusil and avoid those with a high sodium content, such as sodium bicarbonate, if you are aged sixty or older. Also avoid alcohol, coffee, orange juice, and other substances that irritate or increase the amount of acid in your stomach; don't wear tight garments; lose weight; and sleep with the head of your bed raised. Hiatus hernia is very common among people aged sixty or older, but the vast majority of this group have no symptoms (see Chapter 9).

For diverticulosis, a disease that is extremely common among people over sixty, you should avoid laxatives and eat high-fiber foods, especially bran (see Chapter 10). Some older people, however, are sensitive to fiber and roughage, and an excess may cause diarrhea and other distress. Thus, Burkitt's concepts about the benefits of high-fiber diets must be applied with caution to the elderly person, who should experiment to see which foods he or she tolerates best.

According to a study reported in a recent textbook on aging, most of the digestive problems of older people have no organic basis and are largely related to emotional factors. This study of three hundred people over age sixty-five showed that the problems included heartburn, ulcerlike distress, belching, nausea, vomiting, diarrhea, constipation, flatulence, borborygmus, lack of appetite, and weight loss. The main causes of these problems were poor eating and bowel habits, preoccupation with food and elimination, fear of disease and death, and emotional tension and depression related to the problems of growing old.

Older people also have special nutritional needs that are not always met. They often have a poor diet, which can, in turn, affect digestive health. Poor diet in the elderly has many causes, including reduced sensitivity to food odors, and hence to taste, and changes in an older person's perception of food palatability. Because the elderly often have trouble chewing, they are likely to avoid certain necessary foods.

Many older people fear going to the store because the neighborhoods where they have lived and enjoyed security for many years have gradually become high-crime areas. Furthermore, the incomes of many older people are inadequate to meet rising food prices, and this adversely affects eating habits. Finally, many older people lose their desire to eat because of grief, loneliness, and depression. They must cope with retirement, changes in family income, sickness and death among family and friends, and with the prejudices that many older people are subjected to simply because they are old.

PART IV

Taking Care

CHAPTER 13

Professional Service

A DOCTOR once explained why she wanted to become a gastroenterologist when she finished medical school: "It's the only specialty that deals with a system of the body you can see in its entirety without having to cut into it." Thirty years ago, no gastroenterologist could have made this statement. Physicians from the time of William Beaumont had found ways to peer inside the stomach and intestines, and, for the past seventy-five years, had used lighted tubes to do so. But these were stiff and poorly lit hollow metal instruments that were extremely uncomfortable for the patient, and provided limited medical information to the doctor.

During the 1950s, optical engineers developed tiny fibers made of glass or plastic that are as thin, and nearly as flexible, as a human hair. In the earliest application of this technology, as many as one hundred thousand optical fibers were fashioned into medical probes called endoscopes. These optical fibers — the same as those used to improve telephone communications and carry computer services into the home — are extremely efficient light traps that can guide a light beam around the twists and turns of the digestive tract, and have it emerge largely undimmed. About a centimer in diameter and up to six feet long, endoscopes are safer and far more comfortable for patients than the older, inflexible instruments. The endoscope's tip can be bent in any direction, even back upon itself.

Suppose your doctor needs to look at your esophagus and stomach, perhaps to diagnose an inflammation that did not show up on X rays, or to detect an ulcer, or to discover the cause of bleeding from your upper gastrointestinal tract. He or she recommends that you undergo esophagogastroduodenoscopy (EGD, for short). The procedure has another, less intimidating, name: panendoscopy. It is one of the most common procedures in gastroenterology, and can be used to examine all parts of the upper gastrointestinal tract.

The flexible endoscope contains one bundle of fibers that carries light into your innards, and another that carries a color image back to your physician's eye, enabling him or her to spot small areas of disease that the older instruments would have missed. Even modern X rays miss more than one-fourth of all stomach ulcers, especially when there is bleeding or scarring from an ulcer that heals, and then recurs. Panendoscopy is now considered more accurate than X ray in detecting stomach and duodenal ulcers.

Side channels in the flexible endoscope accommodate miniature medical instruments. Among the variety of tools that can be passed through the endoscope channel are forceps and brushes for taking biopsy samples, devices to cauterize tissues, and laser wave-guides. The endoscope also contains a suction channel for removing biopsy samples, and tubes that carry water and air to clean the viewing lens and suspicious areas obscured by blood or mucus.

Snares and forceps can clear a coin from a blocked windpipe, or extract beads, safety pins, and other foreign bodies lodged in the esophagus or stomach. It is a vast improvement over the days when surgeons extracted foreign bodies by having their patients swallow a small sponge on a string, allowing it to moisten and expand in the stomach, and then withdrawing the sponge. This was a favorite technique for removing fish bones. Another crude method of removing a swallowed object was to induce vomiting. Some sharp foreign bodies are still more safely removed by withdrawing them through a rigid esophagoscope. This prevents injury to the esophagus and keeps the foreign body from being inhaled into the airway.

The flexible endoscope's snares and forceps can also snip a tissue sample from the intestine to determine whether it is benign or malignant, cauterize a bleeding ulcer with light from an argon laser, or remove a trapped gallstone, all without major surgery. Other attachments allow doctors to photograph or televise what they have seen. One gastroenterologist used his endoscope to search behind a wall in his house for a leaking pipe. He then sterilized it, of course.

In a feat more fantastic than that accomplished in *Fantastic Voyage*, these forty-inch-long tubes can even snake beyond the small intestine and into the tiny ducts leading from the liver, gallbladder, and pancreas, in order to diagnose cancer and other diseases of these organs. In this new and less commonly used procedure, called endoscopic retrograde cholangiopancreatography, or ERCP, dye injected into the ducts fills the even tinier "upstream" channels and makes them visible by X ray. ERCP has been especially valuable in diagnosing acute pancreatitis, which, for decades, had been detected strictly on the basis of physical examination and medical history. ERCP can be performed only by an extremely skilled endoscopist — as the physicians who specialize in flexible endoscopy are called — and the instrument has limited maneuverability in some areas of the pancreas and biliary duct. You must remain conscious during this thirty- to sixty-minute procedure, but you will be so heavily sedated you probably won't feel anything.

Before you undergo an endoscopy, you will be told not to eat for at least six hours before the test, which can be administered either in a doctor's office or hospital. After you receive a sedative to relax you, and an anesthetic spray to numb your throat, your doctor will ask you to swallow the tube slowly and not to bite. If you gag, your doctor will ask you to breathe slowly around the tube and try to relax. In the hands of a skilled endoscopist, the procedure will not cause undue discomfort, and you can console yourself with the knowledge that, unlike ERCP, it takes about ten minutes, and usually causes no aftereffects.

It is in the lower gastrointestinal tract that fiberoptic instruments have worked the greatest wonders. Colonoscopes about one hundred inches long and the thickness of a thumb can be eased through almost the entire length of the large intestine, completely beyond the range of the rigid proctoscopes, which reach only two feet or so. Colonoscopy can detect the source of hidden bleeding and diagnose pain or other symptoms that X rays cannot conclusively identify. Colonoscopes can also determine the extent of damage caused by ulcerative colitis. They are far more accurate than X rays in detecting precancerous lesions in patients who have had ulcerative colitis for many years. These instruments are also far more accurate than X rays in detecting cancer of the colon.

Perhaps the most valuable contribution of the colonoscope is its utility in the removal of polyps and tumors deep in the intestine. Polyps are growths that range in size from peas to walnuts and hang from the walls of your rectum and colon. Doctors like to remove them because polyps can become cancerous. Using a procedure called endoscopic polypectomy, the endoscope carries a tiny instrument that snips or burns the polyp off. Before this procedure came into use, major surgery was necessary to remove polyps and to biopsy them to determine if they were malignant. With colonoscopy, most polyps can be removed quickly, safely, and painlessly without surgery. And a doctor is more likely to be able to detect a malignancy early using colonoscopy.

Of all the tools gastroenterologists use to diagnose disease, colonoscopy may be the most uncomfortable. You will have to go on a liquid diet for one or two days before the exam and undergo enemas to clean your colon. But the procedure is far less painful and risky than exploratory surgery. Your discomfort can be minimized during the procedure itself if you ask your doctor beforehand for adequate sedation. Colonoscopy usually takes fifteen minutes to an hour and is performed in a hospital as a precaution against emergencies such as perforation and bleeding. The instrument is passed very carefully through the anus and colon. The endoscopist never forces it along. If the doctor has difficulty maneuvering the endoscope around curves in the colon, an X ray can provide information about how to guide it.

Because the field of endoscopy, however promising, is still in its infancy, there are a number of problems and risks entailed. These are minimal when a skilled specialist is performing the procedure. But there is still a serious shortage of trained endoscopists and of adequate facilities to train them. New instruments must be developed to simplify and speed up endoscopic procedures. Colonoscopy, for example, would be a far more widely used procedure if more doctors were expert in it, and if there were instruments that allowed it to be done more quickly.

Until endoscopy becomes more widely used, when your stomach needs testing you are most likely to have an upper gastrointestinal, or "upper GI," series. You must fast for twelve hours before this examination, and somehow manage to swallow a "barium milkshake," which highlights your esophagus, stomach, and small intestine on X rays, and reveals tumors, ulcers, and obstructions, if you have any. The procedure is painless, and the worst part of it is swallowing the barium. You also may have to counteract constipation caused by the barium afterward.

When you have a "lower GI" series, you will be filled with barium from the other end. You must first go on a liquid diet for a day before the exam, and take one or two high-volume (about two thousand milliliters) enemas before the barium itself is injected in your colon in the X ray room. These preparatory enemas are extremely important because, as noted earlier, cancer might be missed during the X ray examination if the colon is not completely cleaned out. Moreover, when feces remain in your colon, they can mimic lesions of the colon, whether caused by ulcerative colitis, polyps, diverticulitis, or cancer. Some studies estimate that as many as seventy-five percent of the cancers of the colon that are missed during X ray examination have been mistaken for or hidden by fecal material. This could mean a fifteen- to twenty-year loss of life because of the resulting delay in surgery for cancer of the colon and rectum.

Two other important tests for diagnosing digestive

problems are computerized axialtomography, also known as the CAT scan, and ultrasonography. CAT scans combine X rays and computer techniques to produce cross-sectional images of the body and its organs. In about forty-five minutes, with no preparation or pain involved, you end up with a full outline of your abdomen and its internal organs. This highly sophisticated machine is as important a medical advance as the discovery of X ray itself.

Ultrasonography, an equally painless procedure, bounces sonar waves off the organs inside your abdomen to detect masses caused by tumors or gallstones. Called "ultrasounds" because humans cannot hear them, these sound waves are particularly valuable in diagnosing liver, biliary tract, and pancreatic diseases because the technique allows careful examination of the interior of solid and fluid-filled body organs without risk to the patient. It even allows examination of the pancreas, once considered a "hidden" organ whose secrets were beyond the reach of X ray and endoscopy. Ultrasound detects pancreatic cysts, tumors, and helps your doctor diagnose both acute and chronic pancreatitis.

Laparoscopy is a test that is not often performed for digestive ailments. It involves cutting a tiny incision through your abdomen near the navel and inserting a nonflexible endoscope to examine the interior of the abdomen. This instrument is the same rigid tube that once was passed down the esophagus to examine the inside of the stomach before flexible endoscopes made their debut. The nonflexible endoscope, called a laparoscope, is used to examine the surface of many of the body's organs — including the liver, gallbladder, spleen, abdominal cavity, and pelvic organs — for tumors and infections. The laparoscope is also used to perform tubal ligations for birth control. Nonflexible endoscopes — while they are largely banned from the upper end of the digestive tract — are still used very successfully in proctoscopy. Proctoscopy, or proctosigmoidoscopy, already described in Chapter 11 as a life-saving examination for cancer of the rectum and colon, is essentially painless if your doctor is skilled, and the embarrassment it entails need last only as long as the test: three to five minutes.

These diagnostic procedures are often more frightening than painful, and are all the more stressful because of your worries about what may be wrong with you. An important part of these procedures, therefore, is to make sure you have a doctor in whom you have confidence. That factor alone can lessen many of the problems — both physical and psychological — that you may have with these tests. In finding a new physician or evaluating your present one, ask yourself these questions:

- Do you and your physician trust one another?
- Does your doctor really listen to you and answer all your questions about the causes, treatment, and prospects for curing your physical problems?
- Is your doctor vague, impatient, or unwilling to answer questions about the nature of your illness and how to deal with it? If so, *find another doctor.*
- Does your doctor take a thorough "history" and ask about your past physical and emotional problems, drugs you are taking, and other matters affecting your health?
- Does your physician seem to automatically prescribe drugs rather than explore the real causes of your medical problems?
- Do you feel free to obtain follow-up information about your illness, its treatment, or a prescription your doctor has given you?
- Does your doctor return phone calls, fit you into his or her schedule when you have an emergency, and provide a colleague to take care of you when he or she is away?
- Does your doctor have adequate experience performing endoscopies or other complicated procedures you must undergo? Ask your doctor how many he or she has done.
- Does your doctor pressure you to have surgery or to refrain from seeking a second opinion about surgery or a major diagnostic test? If so, it may be time to change doctors.

Remember that you are a consumer who is paying for your doctor's services, and that you are entrusting that doctor with your life and your health. You are entitled to ask questions when selecting or dealing with a doctor and to expect reasonable, satisfying answers. Remember, too, that medicine is less a science than an art, and the artist you choose to take care of your body should be the best.

But more than your physician's skill is involved here. A good doctor-patient relationship is based upon mutual respect, open communication, and collaboration and is, in essence, a contract of equals between you and your doctor. He or she should allow you an active role in deciding when to seek medical attention, when to accept or reject medical advice, and when to seek a second opinion from another doctor. However, this does not mean that you should expect your doctor to follow all of your wishes — to prescribe a drug or order a test — unless he or she agrees with the wisdom of that decision. The best doctors are those who, while being flexible and understanding, will not compromise themselves by practicing "bad medicine." You, in turn, owe your physician cooperation and honesty. Above all, you owe yourself a continuing effort to seek the best medical care.

Sometimes this means recognizing that the medical profession, for all its achievements and all its artistry, can do only a certain amount to keep your body and digestion running well. Eighty percent of the general practitioners, family physicians, and internists who treat digestive complaints have received only one month of training in gastrointestinal medicine during four years of medical school. And there are only about four thousand gastroenterologists in the United States available to treat some twenty million people with chronic digestive diseases, let alone the acute, temporary bouts of tummy trouble you have from time to time. This does not mean the medical profession is inadequate to cope with digestive ailments. But it does mean that you should not expect doctors to deal with things you should be doing for yourself. As the poet Alexander Pope once wrote:

> Who shall decide,
> When Doctors disagree . . . ?

CHAPTER 14

Do-It-Yourself
Intestinal Tune-Up

A FEW YEARS AGO, the father of an eminent gastroenterologist refused to undergo an endoscopy. The doctor, in recounting this incident at a medical meeting, said his father recovered anyway. "Eighty-five percent of our patients get well," he added, "no matter what we do."

Most digestive diseases do not kill you, but, like a malfunctioning car, they can keep you from getting around. People with gastrointestinal problems often spend their lives — and their money — checking in and out of hospitals and submitting to repeated surgery and expensive diagnostic tests. Their medicine cabinets, briefcases, and purses too often are crammed with antacids, laxatives, and prescription remedies. Their diseases cause countless emotional and social disruptions and irreversibly alter their lifestyles.

But what if your lifestyle could change your disease? Napoleon Bonaparte, for all his physical and mental endurance, never knew good health. He considered sleep an unfortunate necessity. He could awaken at any hour he previously determined in his mind. He could even doze in the saddle during battle if things were going well. His body, in apparent reaction to the severe treatment he accorded it, contracted pulmonary tuberculosis, cystitis, bladder stones, scabies (little skin-burrowing insects that cause an unbearable itch), epilepsy, and swollen legs. But his stomach was his personal Waterloo. Throughout his life, he suffered frequent intestinal upsets, apparently caused by nervousness and an allergy to cow's milk. He ate strictly to live and derived no enjoyment whatsoever from his meals. He was frequently seized by attacks of severe abdominal pain, probably caused by nervous indigestion, which left him rolling on the ground cursing. Later in life, he had far more serious attacks of what he called "stomach cramps," actually caused by an ulcer. He died, as mentioned in Chapter 9, of perforated ulcer, hemorrhage, and peritonitis. Years of bleeding from the ulcer apparently had caused much of his poor health. Napoleon's ulcer could have been cured today, but the little corporal would have had to shun the tensions of the battlefield and take better care of himself. Both were unlikely events.

For those who are willing to take good care of themselves, there are many ways to bring digestive diseases, particularly minor tummy troubles, under better control. Often such problems can be prevented if you practice self-care. This means being aware of your digestive system and what can go wrong with it, improving your diet and other basic habits, and making healthy changes in your lifestyle. Emotional self-care is perhaps the most important kind of all, since digestive diseases are so clearly identified with the stresses of modern living.

Inner Listening

Instead of telling your stomach to "Shut up!" try listening to it. From time to time, your stomach and other digestive organs send sensory signals that you can hear, see, and feel. Attention to these "inner signals" could eliminate many digestive problems, just as listening to your car's knocks and whines could eliminate many a repair bill. Inner listening also helps you identify "gastroemotional" digestive problems caused by emotional stress. Learn to distinguish the occasional rumbles from the desperate cries for help.

If you are having pains in the chest area, ask yourself:

what type of pain is it? when does it hurt? what makes it worse? Make note of your other symptoms: burping? a searing feeling rising in your throat? These could be signals that you are eating too fast, eating the wrong food, eating at irregular hours, or eating and drinking too much. In short, these signals could mean you have heartburn. If you feel better after trying a mild antacid, switching to simple foods, or eating in an unhurried atmosphere at regular hours, you have diagnosed and cured yourself. If, however, the symptoms continue despite your attempts to remedy them, see a doctor. They could be disguising a more serious condition.

Abdominal pain, another common digestive problem, is not in itself an alarm signal. But when it is accompanied by tenderness, or is very severe, prolonged, or accompanied by persistent diarrhea, chills, or blood and mucus in the stool, all sorts of serious ailments could be involved. Make note of such symptoms as fever, changes in bowel habits, loss of appetite, and unintentional weight loss. They will help your doctor determine what is wrong.

Bowel movements are a visible — if you take care to watch them — sign of your state of health. When they become too loose or too bound, and nothing you do to change your diet helps, the problem should be reported to your physician. Too often, bowel disorders are mistreated with enemas, laxatives, and other chemical bowel regulators.

Learn to distinguish sensible health practices from those which are nonsense. This includes knowing which drugs and patent remedies to avoid, which to take, and when to take them. The taboos that surround constipation, hemorrhoids, and other colon and rectal disorders feed a thriving industry that pushes patent medicine remedies and "cures" that may — if improperly used — prolong suffering and delay needed medical care. In too many cases, the cost of such delay is life itself. Heavily advertised laxatives, antacids, and hemorrhoid remedies are among the worst offenders. Even when a drug is prescribed by a doctor, that does not necessarily mean it is effective. In early 1981, for example, the Food and Drug Administration proposed stopping the sale of eighteen combination drugs that doctors had been prescribing for gastrointestinal disorders. The proposal was the first step in removing the drugs from the market. See Chapter 15 for a list of nonprescription drugs that can safely be included in the home pharmacy for constipation, diarrhea, hemorrhoids, and other "stomach" ailments.

Healthful Habits

You can also take steps to keep stomach troubles from occurring or getting worse. These measures include maintaining a well-balanced diet, getting exercise, and successfully handling emotional stress. The kind of food you eat, for example, has profound effects on your digestive tract, which uses, detoxifies, and disposes of what you eat. Indeed, diet is one factor you *can* control that directly contributes to digestive health or illness. Consider: hiatus hernia, gallbladder disease, appendicitis, diverticular disease, hemorrhoids, and cancer of the colon and rectum have only in recent decades become health problems in the United States and other modern Western nations. Yet, in other areas of the world where people have not yet adopted American-style eating habits and highly processed foods, these conditions are rare or unheard of. These diseases may be related to the amount of fiber in your diet, which is related to the bulk and consistency of stools, which, in turn, affects the amount of time it takes food to pass through the digestive tract. From the health standpoint, the shorter the transit time, the better. Thus, many physicians and nutritional experts believe that a well-balanced diet that is high in fiber provides protection against many of these diseases and makes sound physiological sense.

There are some problems with fiber that should be mentioned. The least serious is that it can temporarily cause flatulence when undigested fiber is attacked by bacteria in the large intestine. A more serious problem is that fiber can deplete your body's supply of certain nutrients, including calcium, zinc, iron, magnesium, phosphorus, and copper, and can keep your body from absorbing dietary protein. Most people have an excess of these nutrients to start with, or manage to adapt to the altered balance. However, people with border-line nutrition such as many of the elderly, or people who have diabetes and other serious diseases, should not switch to fiber unless their physicians advise it. It is best to add fiber to your diet gradually — eat a variety of high-fiber foods rather than concentrating on just one, and drink lots of liquids so the fiber won't become constipating (see Appendix C).

It also makes sound physiological sense to avoid harmful substances such as excessive alcohol, aspirin, cigarette smoke, and, perhaps, coffee. There is a phrase in the computer world that might be applied to the inner world of digestion: garbage in, garbage out.

Exercise is a prime way to prevent constipation. It also helps keep you from becoming obese, which can undermine your digestive and general health. Pot bellies, for example, are charming on stoves, but not on people. A flat belly supports and protects the abdominal organs, including the liver, gallbladder, and stomach. Strong abdominals help the body to vomit when necessary and stimulate peristalsis or intestinal activity by causing pressure against the large bowel. There are many ways you can strengthen your abdominal muscles, which, in people with sedentary lifestyles, are too often underexercised. You can do an isometric exercise in which you stand or sit up straight, take a deep breath, pull in your abdominal muscles while slowly exhaling for a count of ten, and then relax. Do ten repetitions of this exercise several times during the day — in elevators, at your desk, or while stopping for traffic lights. Some doctors prescribe an exercise program consisting of sit-ups, leg-raises, toe-touches, side-bends and back-bends. Good exercise technique involves doing each exercise slowly and rhythmically, stopping if it causes pain, and never holding your breath while exercising.

Reducing disruptive emotional stresses in your life can also help you digest food better and keep your intestinal tract in tune. Learn how to recognize situations that create unpleasant or frightening feelings, and how to express these feelings directly rather than through your gut. Stress, per se, is neither harmful nor beneficial. How you handle it is another matter entirely. For some people, a stressful situation — such as giving an after-dinner speech or competing for a promotion — spurs them on to better performance. For others, a stressful situation leaves them feeling unhinged. You might try these techniques for coping with negative stress:

- Learn how to say no.
- Recognize situations that cause stress for you.
- Recognize the symptoms of stress.
- Avoid crutches like food, drugs, or alcohol for coping with stress.
- Set attainable goals.
- Tackle stressful projects one step at a time.
- Learn how to talk out problems with the people involved.
- Exercise regularly to let off steam.
- Never use illness to gain sympathy or attention.

Because these are not skills many people automatically possess, it is sometimes necessary to get some help from books, from friends who have learned some of these techniques and, best of all, from psychiatrists, psychologists, social workers, clergymen, and other professionals. Millions of men and women who have sought help are not insane or irrational or even flaky. They are anxious, depressed, and unwilling to get mired down in ill-health and unhappiness.

How well they do in psychotherapy depends upon how much effort — and money — they are willing to spend. Success also depends upon selecting the right therapist with the right skills, with whom it is possible to develop a trusting relationship. This relationship is what makes the process succeed or fail. There are two kinds of psychotherapy: short-term, which helps you with immediate crises such as divorce, death, or loss of a job; and long-term, which continues for a number of years and is advisable when problems — including health problems for which a physical cause cannot be found — tend to occur over and over again. Then it is helpful to explore the emotions that underlie these problems, for this helps you modify behavior patterns that are self-defeating. Therapy may be on a one-to-one basis if the emphasis is on exploring your past and its effect on present-day behavior. Or your problems may better be handled in a group of five to eight other patients, especially if you have trouble relating to others. Many times, you are advised to combine both kinds of therapy. The cost per fifty-minute session ranges from $35 to $60 or more in some cities. Group therapy is somewhat less expensive. Unfortunately, health insurance picks up very little of the tab.

Because psychotherapy entails so much expense and personal effort, you should take great care in choosing a therapist:

♦ Shop around. Ask respected friends (or your family physician or minister) for a referral.

♦ When you visit a therapist for the first few times, remember that these are exploratory visits, not commitments to return for treatment. Indeed, you can stop therapy at any time, but you owe yourself a good look at your reasons for doing so.

♦ At the outset, discuss fees and the time of your regular appointment and explore the therapist's background and values.

♦ During the first several visits, state what you expect to gain from therapy, and ask for the therapist's estimate of how long your treatment program should continue.

♦ If, for any reason, you feel uncomfortable with the therapist, find another one. But remember that if you change therapists three or four times, the problem may lie with you, not with them.

♦ Expect, over the long run, a sense of progress and relief, despite the emotional discomfort of therapy.

Therapists have a saying, "You will feel a lot worse before you feel better." This refers to the fact that during the early stages of psychotherapy, long-repressed feelings and emotional conflicts come to the surface and can cause you conscious pain. But the same feelings, when denied, can express themselves in such unhealthy ways as constipation, ulcers, irritable bowel syndrome, and a host of digestive and other illnesses. For people who don't believe that psychological stresses have any bearing on digestive or any other kinds of disease — but who cannot find any physical causes for their ailments — it cannot hurt to explore the emotional side.

Whether you have learned to recognize and express your feelings, or simply to relax when they get you down, you emerge from therapy with a sense of being able to do something about a physical problem. One technique that can relieve your feelings of helplessness and anxiety is biofeedback. This is a way of controlling and stabilizing your body's physical and emotional reactions. For example, you can learn to exert voluntary control over your skin temperature, heart rate, blood pressure, muscle tension, brain waves, or any other body function that can be monitored. A special type of muscle biofeedback has enabled many people to control tension headaches, asthma, menstrual distress, and intestinal disorders such as colitis and spasms of the smooth muscles of the intestines. In one study, subjects with diarrhea, for which no physical cause could be found, were asked to listen to the amplified sounds of peristaltic activity in their overactive guts. The sounds were picked up through an electronic stethoscope, amplified, and played back through a loudspeaker. The subjects were then asked to increase or decrease their intestinal activity, and were verbally encouraged each time they succeeded. With only five training sessions lasting thirty minutes each, all of them were able to control bowel motility to some degree. A group of patients with irritable bowel syndrome (mentioned in Chapter 10) were able, with the help of doctors at The Johns Hopkins Hospital in Baltimore, to suppress colon spasms whenever they saw them recorded on a piece of paper.

In other gastrointestinal applications of biofeedback, people have learned to control fecal incontinence, esophageal spasms, vomiting, and gastric acid secretion. In this last experiment, patients swallowed a pH electrode that was connected to a meter that gave them visual feedback on how much gastric acid they were secreting. They were then asked to control these secretions. In one variation, a subject was asked to increase gastric acid secretion by thinking of gourmet foods, and to decrease it by thinking about nonfood items. Biofeedback is mentioned in this self-help chapter because although you need a biofeedback therapist to learn it, the success of the technique is completely up to you. You are no longer a body being acted upon by the medical profession. It is you, not the doctor or therapist, who possesses the power to rid your body of certain biological reactions that can cause pain and disease. In essence, you observe what your body is doing and change it. Eventually, you learn to control headache, diarrhea, or other physical problems *without* the biofeedback signal. Then you, not the diarrhea, are in control.

Another, more controversial, self-help technique is "imaging," in which you picture a desired outcome and allow expectations of illness or health to provide a way to regulate the course of a disease. For example, in regular exercises, you might visualize cancer cells in your body as little frightened fish that are destroyed by white blood cells that look like voracious sharks. Thus, you accentuate the positive and eliminate the negative in a technique that is based upon the principles of psychotherapy. Perhaps the most important aspect of biofeedback and imaging is that you acknowledge your participation in the onset of disease and, therefore, your power to regain or maintain your health.

The best ways to take charge of your health are often very simple. Consider this story of a man who had been under enormous stress for several months:

> When I realized I wasn't enjoying my food, and that I was just eating it, I psyched myself into enjoying my meals. Then, one day, I had a brainstorm: why not enjoy *digesting* as well as eating my food? I decided to take five to ten minutes after every meal to do just that. When I tried it, I actually got a good feeling in my tummy and it felt like I was helping the digestive process. Then I asked myself the ultimate question: 'Why not enjoy eliminating it too?'

This book goes one step further to ask: if you don't enjoy as basic a pleasure as eating — and the body processes that go along with it — and in that way, take good care of yourself, who will?

CHAPTER 15

Trouble-Shooter's Guide

LEROY ROBERT (SATCHEL) PAIGE, one of the all-time great baseball pitchers, once advised, "If your stomach disputes you, lie down and pacify it with cool thoughts." Here, for convenience, is a summary of the practical advice offered in earlier pages. When stomach disputes send you back to this book to refresh your memory at a later date, you may find it easier to have "cool thoughts" about your ailment listed in alphabetical order in the pages that follow. If you are suffering from constipation, for example, you will find home remedies for it listed under "C." Advice for self-care of ulcers is listed last, under "U."

This advice is *not* meant to substitute for professional medical care, but is a trouble-shooting guide to help you take the best possible care of your stomach. Each section, which contains advice about what to do if you have heartburn, constipation, intestinal gas, or some more serious condition: 1) briefly describes symptoms that will help you recognize whether you have a problem; 2) lists things you can do to prevent or relieve it; and 3) tells you when to stop trying to treat yourself and see a doctor. For example, any time you

have abdominal pain accompanied by tenderness, very severe pain, pain lasting longer than six hours, or recurring
pain that you cannot explain, call a doctor. Other serious
warning signals that could indicate any number of serious
digestive disorders requiring a physician's attention include:

- Sudden change in bowel habits.
- Bloody, black, or gray stools.
- Blood in vomitus.
- Fever lasting longer than two days, or over 101 de-
  grees.
- Loss of weight or appetite.
- Jaundice (yellowed skin and whites of the eyes)
- Pain or difficulty swallowing food.

Fortunately, most digestive disorders are not serious or
life-threatening. But they are often painful, emotionally upsetting, expensive to treat, and disruptive to your everyday
life. And, unless you know how to prevent and take care of
these disorders, they will tend to recur again and again.

Appendicitis The symptoms of an inflamed appendix are
familiar: sudden, sharp pain around the navel, which grows
worse and, in a few hours, shifts to the lower right (or sometimes the left) side of your abdomen. The pain may intensify
if you press on your lower right side or move your right leg.
You may become nauseated or vomit. Your fever may climb
to 102°F., and a child's fever may soar even higher.

Symptoms are not always predictable. You may simply
have persistent abdominal pain, while a young child may
experience nothing more than vomiting, fever, and irritability. If the pain lasts longer than three to four hours, call a
doctor, for you may be in danger of a ruptured appendix.

Appendicitis is one problem you should not self-treat.
Home remedies like heating pads, cathartics, and enemas can
obscure symptoms, intensify intestinal contractions, and may
even cause your appendix to rupture.

Belching About belching, first cousin to intestinal gas, it
can only be said:

It's better to belch,
And bear the shame,
Than squelch a belch,
And bear the pain!

Borborygmus Also known as musical stomach, this perfectly normal sound of air and liquid from digesting food sloshing around inside your stomach and intestines is best quelled when you:

♦ Lie down on your back or your right side and apply pressure to your abdomen.
♦ Avoid carbonated beverages.
♦ Eat something. Although borborygmus is not caused by hunger, per se, the anticipation of eating can generate borborygmic rumblings.
♦ Remember that air swallowing contributes to borborygmus, and nervousness contributes to air swallowing.
♦ Don't be embarrassed when you hear a stomach growl, whether it's yours or somebody else's. Tell the audience to enjoy the stomach's concert.

High-pitched sounds mean air or fluid is moving under high pressure through a narrow passage such as the small intestine. Low-pitched rumbles mean air and fluid are going through a large passage under low pressure.

Cancer of the Digestive Tract No disease provokes such widespread fear as cancer, partly because many people do not realize that great progress has been made against the disease. An estimated fifty percent of all cancer patients in the United States could live the rest of their lives without a recurrence of their cancer if they took advantage of currently available diagnostic and treatment techniques.

For example, cancers of the colon and rectum can be cured if detected early enough. Yet many tumors of the large bowel still go undetected. Therefore, if you are over the age of forty, the American Cancer Society (ACS) recommends an annual physical and digital examination in which your physician inserts a gloved finger into your rectum to detect any cancerous areas just inside the anus. If you are over the age of fifty, the ACS also recommends an annual proctosigmoidoscopic or "procto" exam. A physician inserts a lighted tube into the first twelve inches of your rectum and lower colon to look for tumors and other abnormalities. The test only takes about five minutes, and is worth the minor discomfort, for cancers detected by digital and "procto" exams have a high cure rate.

For the over-fifty group, the ACS also recommends that you conduct a test at home once a year to detect hidden blood in your stool since most colon cancers cause abnormal bleeding. You simply eat a meat-free, high-fiber diet for at least forty-eight hours or until you have collected specimens from three consecutive stools. These specimens are placed on a special paper slide that can detect the presence of blood. Give this slide to your physician, who will have it evaluated and report the results to you.

Many people in whom cancer has been detected do not take advantage of the best treatments medicine has to offer. Many others do not avoid known causes of cancer, such as smoking, and do not adopt healthful practices, such as a high-fiber and low-fat diet, that appear to prevent cancer. And many people do not know whether they are in a high-risk group for cancer of the colon, liver, or some other organ. For example, individuals with ulcerative colitis for ten years or longer are at high risk for cancer of the colon, and people who carry the hepatitis B virus appear to be at higher risk for liver cancer.

Regardless of your risk status, you should know the warning signs of cancer:

- Severe pain lasting longer than six hours, unexplained pain, or mild pain lasting longer than two weeks.
- Sudden changes in bowel habits.
- Bright red or black blood in your stool.
- Blood in vomitus.
- Gray or clay-colored stools.
- Persistent or recurring fever of 101°F. or higher.
- Sudden loss of weight or appetite.

♦ Jaundice or dark urine.
♦ Difficulty swallowing food.

If any of these symptoms occur, see your doctor immediately.

Celiac Disease and Lactose Intolerance Inability to digest gluten or milk can cause digestive problems in young children and, in some cases, adults. Abdominal pain, gas, bloating, and foul-smelling diarrhea containing undigested food particles are among the symptoms of inability to digest gluten (celiac disease) or milk (lactose intolerance). The remedy for celiac disease is to avoid eating foods containing wheat, oats, barley, buckwheat, and rye. People with lactose intolerance need not avoid milk and milk products entirely, just to the degree necessary to ease symptoms.

The completely intolerant must eliminate all dairy products, including sugar substitutes containing lactose. Read labels carefully.

Cirrhosis of the Liver This disease — and a number of other serious liver disorders — may cause you to lose weight, suffer stomach upsets, vomit, and have trouble digesting fats. If the disease has progressed — and often it has before you or your doctor discovers it — your skin and eyes may turn a yellowish color, and you may pass dark urine. Your skin may itch and spidery blood vessels may appear on your face and neck. You may have abdominal pain and swelling, and you may vomit blood or pass it in your stools — these symptoms indicate intestinal bleeding. If you are male, as most cirrhotics are, your breasts may enlarge and irreversible impotence may occur.

The remedy for cirrhosis of the liver—a hardening of that organ into scar tissue, which is usually caused by excessive alcohol consumption over a period of many years—is quite simple. Although cirrhosis, or scarring of your liver, cannot be reversed, it can be slowed down and even stopped. All it takes is quitting the booze.

Prolonged exposure to environmental toxins can also cause cirrhosis. When using chemicals at home, at work, or in your garden, the American Liver Foundation recommends that you:

♦ Make sure there is good ventilation.
♦ Follow directions on the label.
♦ Never mix chemical products.
♦ Don't get chemicals on your skin. If you do, wash them off immediately because they can be absorbed.
♦ Do not inhale chemicals, and wear protective clothing when using them.

You should also learn to recognize the symptoms of liver disease:

♦ Jaundice (yellowed skin and whites of eyes).
♦ Dark urine.
♦ Gray or light-colored stools.
♦ Nausea and vomiting or blood.
♦ Black or bloody stools.
♦ Loss of appetite.
♦ Abdominal swelling and pain.
♦ Prolonged itching all over the body.
♦ Unusual change in weight.
♦ Fatigue and loss of stamina.
♦ Sleep disturbances.
♦ Mental confusion or coma.

Colic One of the first, and most common, digestive distresses of infants aged one to three months is colic, or sharp intestinal pain caused by the muscular waves and contractions of the stomach. The underlying cause appears to be tension and fatigue rather than diet. To keep colic under control:

♦ Keep yourself and your baby calm.
♦ Lay the baby, stomach down, over your knees or over a hot water bottle wrapped in a towel.
♦ Try riding with the baby in a car, rocking, or swinging the baby gently in a mechanical swing.

If colic is severe or you feel unable to deal with it, see your pediatrician.

Constipation   Many people think they are constipated when they really are not. Constipation is a problem *not* when your bowels fail to move, but when you feel mild pain and discomfort *because* your bowels have not moved.

You seldom need drugs or a doctor to treat constipation. All you need do is:

♦ Eat a high-fiber diet consisting of fruits, vegetables, whole-grain cereals and bread, and bran. This diet is the foremost remedy for constipation.
♦ Take a "daily constitutional," or start swimming, bicycling, gardening, or engaging in some other activity.
♦ If diet and exercise don't work, try a bulk laxative such as Metamucil or Effersylium.
♦ Drink lots of fluids: eight to ten full glasses daily.
♦ Try prune juice. It contains a chemical that gets the gut moving.
♦ Eat breakfast or drink a cup of coffee or something warm, also to get things moving.
♦ For babies, it often helps to add a teaspoon or two of corn syrup to their formula, or to give them prune juice or stewed prunes. For older children, the remedies are the same as for adults.
♦ Avoid repeated use of laxatives, mineral oil, and enemas. They create the problem they were meant to cure and they can damage the bowel reflex, become habit-forming, and interfere with other digestive processes.

As long as you are comfortable and can pass even a hard, dry stool easily, it doesn't matter how often stool passes. You should see a doctor, however, if constipation occurs suddenly or is accompanied by severe abdominal cramps and bloating, pitch black stools or the passage of blood, or pencillike or ribbonlike stools.

Diarrhea   Whether you call diarrhea the trots, the runs, the green apple quick-step, Montezuma's revenge, "turista," or Delhi belly, the symptoms range from occasional loose stools to profuse, watery diarrhea and cramping abdominal pain.

If you're down with diarrhea:

◆ Get plenty of physical rest.

◆ Avoid solid foods and drink warm liquids (tea, broth, water, and flat soda) to replace fluids and salts lost through diarrhea.

◆ Drink fluids containing sugar and salt, such as Gatorade or a home mixture of ½ teaspoon table salt, ½ teaspoon baking soda, ¼ teaspoon potassium chloride, and 2 tablespoons glucose. You may need a physician's prescription for the potassium chloride.

◆ As long as you feel dehydrated, the more you drink of this mixture, the better.

◆ Drink liquids between meals rather than with them.

◆ As your condition improves, add soups, Jell-O, applesauce, and bland foods like rice and toast.

◆ Replace potassium, which is depleted when you have diarrhea, by eating bananas, potatoes, meat, and fish, or ask your doctor about potassium supplements.

◆ Avoid milk and high-fiber foods like fruits and vegetables with seeds and tough skins until your intestines calm down.

◆ Don't eat foods that are fatty, spicy, or that cause gas or cramps. These include carbonated drinks, beer, beans, cabbage, cauliflower, sweets, and chewing gum.

◆ Work up slowly to a normal diet.

◆ If these measures do not work, try a tablespoon of Kaopectate after each loose bowel movement.

◆ If Kaopectate does not work, try paregoric, a narcotic that slows down the digestive tract. Parapectolin and Parelixir may be available without a prescription.

◆ Lomotil, a prescription drug, may temporarily relieve diarrhea but should be used with caution since it can lead to dependency and, in some cases, can prolong rather than cure the problem.

If diarrhea lasts longer than seventy-two hours, if it has blood in it, or if you have severe abdominal pain, see a doctor.

Many cases of diarrhea occur when you are traveling. To prevent "turista":

◆ Learn about food and water safety in the places you will visit, and where to go for medical help.

◆ Avoid exposure to unsafe water, including ice cubes in drinks, lettuce and fruit washed in unsafe water, milk, and frozen confections sold by street venders.

◆ Boil the water that you use for drinking and for brushing your teeth with an electric immersion coil, or treat it with water purification tablets.

◆ Avoid poolside smorgasbords and buffets and, when swimming, keep your mouth shut.

◆ While abroad, don't get physically run down and don't go on eating binges.

◆ Wash your hands frequently and thoroughly. Many travelers peel their oranges with contaminated hands and wonder why they get turista!

Diverticulosis This disease is characterized by the presence of many pouches protruding outward from the lining of the colon wall. These sacs can trap fecal material as it passes by. Most people who have diverticulosis do not even know it. Symptoms, if they occur, include gas, stomach cramps, and diarrhea alternating with constipation. Pain on the lower left side of the abdomen may occur at evening mealtime, when the gut is most active.

About fifteen percent of people with diverticulosis develop diverticu*litis*, an infection of one or more sacs in the colon wall. Symptoms include a steady, severe pain in your left side that hurts more if you press down on that area. The pain may last minutes or days, and may be accompanied by fever, chills, gas pains, constipation, or alternating diarrhea and constipation.

Diverticulitis requires a physician's care. You will probably be treated with bed rest, heat over your left side, a low-fiber diet with clear fluids to rest your bowel, stool softeners, and antibiotics to clear the inflammation. After symptoms subside, you will go on a very soft diet, and gradually transfer to a high-fiber diet. Most people can control the underlying problem, diverticulosis, by avoiding laxatives and cathartics, and by eating high-fiber foods, especially bran. However, older people are sometimes sensitive to fiber, and sudden or excessive amounts may cause diarrhea and other distresses.

Gallbladder Disease Some twenty million Americans have gallstones — clumps of fat that collect in the gallbladder. They may lie there quietly, but sometimes they migrate and temporarily get stuck in the narrow ducts leading from the gallbladder to the small intestine. When this happens, you may feel faintness, nausea, chills, indigestion, or pain resembling a stitch in the side. The pain can be so intense that you vomit, become wet with perspiration, and perhaps develop fever and chills, usually within one to two hours after eating a rich, fatty meal. The attack may last a few minutes or a week. If you experience these symptoms, call a doctor.

If a gallstone permanently lodges in the bile duct, it will prevent bile produced by the liver from reaching your intestine. This, in turn, causes jaundice, light gray or white stools (because bile is what turns your stools dark), and tea- or cola-colored urine. Some cases of gallstone blockage respond to nonsurgical treatment such as cutting down on fatty foods, but the usual cure is removal of the gallbladder.

Halitosis Halitosis (bad breath) or *fetor oris* (*very* bad breath) may originate in your lungs, breathing passages, or nose. But eighty-five to ninety percent of "bird cage breath" originates in your mouth. Most cases of halitosis can be avoided if you:

◆ Brush your teeth, gums, and tongue as far back as possible three times daily. A coated tongue, especially the back portion, which emits the strongest odor, can cause bad breath.

◆ Avoid breathing through your mouth. Dry mouth and mouth breathing also cause foul breath because saliva cannot wash your mouth free of bacteria and their smelly by-products.

◆ Suck sugarless lozenges to help increase the flow of saliva between tooth brushings.

◆ Visit your dentist regularly to have decay-causing plaque (invisible bacterial accumulations on the teeth) removed, and control it between visits by brushing, and flossing between the teeth.

◆ Do not use mouthwashes. They do little more than mask halitosis for a few hours.

◆ Eat. However, as Shakespeare advises in *A Midsummer Night's Dream* (act 4, scene 2, line 40): "Eat no onions nor garlic, for we are to utter sweet breath."

◆ Avoid high-fat foods (especially milk and butter fats), refined sugar, and white flour if you are prone to halitosis.

Hangovers Hangovers — also known as the sobering-up syndrome — are the price people pay for drinking too much. The tab usually includes a monstrous headache, dehydration, nausea, dizziness, fatigue, and a feeling of general malaise.

The best remedy for hangovers is to avoid getting them:

◆ Relax or nap before a party. Fatigue increases the rate of alcohol absorption in your body. Fear, anger and sadness have the same effect.

◆ Eat dinner before a party. Food slows the rate at which you absorb alcohol.

◆ Allow time between drinks so that you don't exceed one containing an ounce of eighty-proof alcohol, or one can of beer, or 3½ ounces of table wine per hour.

◆ Use water rather than soda as a mixer.

◆ Know how medications you are taking interact with alcohol. For example, some cough and cold remedies can heighten the effects of alcohol.

The best remedy for a hangover is rest and the passage of time, and the next best is to combat dehydration:

◆ Before retiring, drink several glasses of water along with something to eat that's salty, like soda crackers.

◆ When you wake up, drink a salt solution such as Gatorade or tomato juice, or drink water and eat soda crackers. Then go back to bed while the salt solution rehydrates your body.

◆ Do not take "hair-of-the-dog-that-bit-you" remedies for hangovers. More liquor the morning after may deaden immediate symptoms for a while, but it also can lead to alcohol dependency.

♦ Avoid mild tranquilizers, sedatives, and antihistamines because they, like alcohol, are depressants that make a hangover worse.

♦ Aspirin may relieve a hangover headache, but it can also irritate your stomach. So can a cup of coffee. Take aspirin with a large glass of water to dilute its corrosive effect.

♦ Do not combine alcohol and aspirin. They are believed to harm the stomach more, when taken together, than either substance does when taken alone.

Heartburn Heartburn is characterized by a steady, burning pain at the tip of your breastbone that occurs when your stomach is full. The pain may travel into your arms. It usually strikes thirty minutes to two hours after a meal, and is made worse by lying down.

How to handle heartburn:

♦ Sit up or stand after eating until gravity settles "acids" back into your stomach.

♦ Sleep with your head raised at least four inches.

♦ Avoid food and drink for two hours before going to bed.

♦ Avoid alcohol, aspirin, coffee, tea, and smoking.

♦ Eat smaller portions of food, increasing the number of meals if necessary.

♦ Avoid milk. It increases gastric secretions and does not help heartburn.

♦ Take nonabsorbable antacids like Maalox or Mylanta about an hour after meals and at bedtime, or more often if symptoms persist.

♦ Do not use sodium bicarbonate or high sodium antacids like Alka-Seltzer and Bromo-Seltzer repeatedly. Avoid them completely if you have heart disease or high blood pressure.

♦ Liquid antacids coat the stomach better than tablets, which must be chewed well to be effective.

♦ Chill liquid antacids. They taste better that way.

♦ Try to correct "heartburn habits" like belching, swallowing air, chewing gum, sucking on hard candies, eating too fast, eating too much, slumping on a full stomach, and taking naps after meals.

See a doctor immediately if heartburnlike pain occurs after exercising and if, in addition, you have trouble swallowing food, are vomiting black or bloody material, passing bloody or tarlike black stools, or feeling "heartburn" pain clear through to your back.

Hemorrhoids Hemorrhoids, or piles, are enlarged veins in your rectum or in the muscular tissues of the anus. They may cause no problem at all. But when they enlarge, they may bleed from the rectum or visibly protrude through your anus, causing itching, burning, discharge, pain during bowel movements, and pain in the rectal area.

Many hemorrhoid sufferers sit on their problem (sitting, in fact, helps produce it) rather than seek medical treatment.

To relieve hemorrhoids:

♦ Apply zinc oxide paste or powder to external hemorrhoids.

♦ Relieve external and internal hemorrhoids with hot baths, aspirin, stool softeners such as Metamucil, bed rest in a prone position, and an ice bag on the anus to relieve pain.

♦ Keep the anal area clean with toilet paper moistened with water or with your own saliva.

♦ It sometimes helps to apply direct finger pressure (with a clean finger) to push a prolapsed pile back into your rectum.

♦ Before using an over-the-counter hemorrhoid remedy, make sure the anal area is clean or you will trap bacteria beneath.

♦ In general, commercial hemorrhoid preparations are of debatable value, and should never become a substitute for proper medical care, or a way of avoiding the embarrassment of admitting you have piles.

♦ Do not use commercial hemorrhoid products on children under twelve years old.

In general, hemorrhoids that cause no symptoms should be left alone. Even bleeding from hemorrhoids — evidenced by bright red blood on the stool or on toilet paper — is not medically significant unless it continues for several weeks. If hemorrhoids cause itching, burning, pain, bleeding, or remain protruded from your anus for longer than a week, see a doctor.

The best way to prevent hemorrhoids is to lose weight, exercise regularly, avoid prolonged standing and sitting, avoid excessive straining at stool, drink lots of fluids to prevent constipation, avoid laxatives, and eat a balanced diet containing fiber. Many a hemorrhoid sufferer has discovered that dietary measures alone will solve the problem.

Hepatitis The other major liver disease is hepatitis, an inflammation of the liver usually caused by viruses (although alcohol, certain drugs, and chemicals in the environment can cause it, too). At least three different types of viral hepatitis have been identified: hepatitis A, hepatitis B, and, for lack of a better name, non-A, non-B (NANB) hepatitis. The symptoms are similar for all three: nausea, weakness, loss of appetite, headache, and flulike fever. In more severe cases, you may develop profound fatigue, pain, and tenderness in your upper right side, jaundice (yellowing of the skin and whites of the eyes), and dark orange-brown urine. The treatment is rest and the passage of time.

Since hepatitis A virus is transmitted by contact with an infected person's feces, the best way to prevent this disease is good sanitation:

♦ Avoid potentially contaminated food and water.
♦ Meticulously wash your hands after going to the bathroom and before eating.
♦ Avoid intimate physical contact with infected people, with their body fluids, and with their food and eating utensils.
♦ Remember that hepatitis A can also be transmitted sexually through oral-anal contact or anal intercourse.

♦ If you have been exposed to hepatitis A, ask your doctor about an injection of immune serum globulin, a blood protein that helps provide immunity for three to four months. The sooner you have this injection after exposure, the better.

♦ Immune serum globulin shots are strongly recommended for travelers to countries where sanitation is poor.

Hepatitis B virus is a far more serious infection. It can lead to lingering liver disease and causes about ten percent of those who contract it to become carriers capable of passing the disease on to others. The hepatitis B virus is spread through blood or other body fluids such as breast milk, saliva, and semen. Injections with hepatitis B immune globulin (HBIG) may help prevent hepatitis B infections in people who have been exposed, and a hepatitis B vaccine has recently been licensed.

People who are known carriers of hepatitis B infection should:

♦ Never share any items that may puncture the skin or become contaminated with body fluids. These include razor blades, scissors, nail files, needles, toothbrushes, and enema or douche equipment.

♦ Never donate blood.

♦ Abstain from kissing and sexual contact while the disease is active.

♦ Cover cuts and sores to avoid exposing others.

♦ Tell your doctor and dentist, laboratory technicians, and others who may draw blood or perform surgical procedures about your disease.

♦ Tell family members and other intimates to see a physician.

Non-A, non-B (NANB) hepatitis is often spread by blood transfusion. Unfortunately, no blood test yet can reliably detect carriers. They usually are discovered only when the blood they donate infects a recipient. Carriers should follow the same precautions as those listed above for persons with hepatitis B.

Hiatus Hernia   Many people who have hiatus hernia do not even know it. But when pressures from the stomach are stronger than the esophageal valve at the entrance to the stomach, the valve may allow digestive juices to back into the esophagus, or tube through which food passes into the stomach. These juices will attack the sensitive mucous membrane lining the walls of the esophagus and cause severe heartburn — the burning pain, pressure, and sour regurgitation that usually strike within a half-hour after a meal. Or the lining of the esophagus may become inflamed and produce pains so sharp that some people confuse them with heart disease.

These complications of hiatus hernia need not occur if you give heartburn and esophagitis "careful handling" at the outset:

- Take antacids as prescribed by your doctor to neutralize stomach acids and reduce inflammation of the esophagus.
- Avoid foods and other substances that compound the problem: alcohol, aspirin, coffee, tea, milk, chocolate, garlic, onion, highly spiced and fatty foods, and peppermint.
- Lose weight if you are too heavy.
- Sleep with the head of your bed raised four to ten inches.
- Eat smaller meals more frequently, and don't eat until you feel stuffed.
- Don't smoke, especially if you have "smoker's cough."
- Don't go to bed on a full stomach.
- Don't exercise immediately after eating.
- Don't wear tight clothes.
- Avoid sudden physical exertion and don't bend forward to scrub floors or weed the garden.
- Remember that the problems that accompany hiatus can be triggered by coughing, vomiting, straining at stool, pregnancy, and obesity, all of which exert pressure on the stomach and abdomen.
- Emotional stress can also aggravate these problems since tension increases the secretion of gastric juices.

♦ Correct "heartburn habits" and follow the heartburn precautions listed earlier.

If heartburn and other problems caused by hiatus hernia don't respond to these common-sense measures, see your doctor. Neglect of these conditions could lead to scarring and narrowing of the esophagus, and possibly even to an inability to swallow solid food.

Hiccups There are many remedies for hiccups. Here are a few:

♦ Hold your breath.
♦ Drink water.
♦ Breathe into a paper bag.
♦ Have somebody frighten you.
♦ Drink water by sipping from the far side of the glass.
♦ Swallow with a pencil between your teeth.
♦ Tickle your nose until you sneeze, or pull out your tongue, or make yourself vomit. (These remedies work because they interrupt the reflex that causes hiccups.)
♦ Swallow a teaspoonful of white granulated sugar dry.

When hiccups last longer than a few hours or recur with frequency, you should see a doctor because more elaborate medical treatment may be necessary. This is unusual, however. For most people, an attack of hiccups is over in less than an hour.

Ileitis or Crohn's Disease This is a severe and chronic inflammation of the deeper layers of the wall of the small intestine, although it may involve the large intestine as well. The disease causes severe abdominal pain, usually in the lower right side. Diarrhea may occur up to twenty times a day, and is often accompanied by blood, pus, and large amounts of mucus. Crohn's disease also may cause intestinal abnormalities, malnutrition, liver disorders, and serious diseases of other parts of the body. When the disease occurs during childhood or early adolescence, it may retard growth and sexual development. In some cases, growth failure is for years the only evidence of this bowel disease in children.

Treatment—which must be under a physician's supervision—consists mainly of controlling symptoms such as pain and bowel activity. This is accomplished with powerful drugs that can cause undesirable side effects. Often prolonged hospitalization and repeated surgery are necessary because Crohn's disease tends to recur.

Indigestion Probably the most common digestive complaint, indigestion ranges from mild discomfort in the midriff area after a meal, to a bloated feeling, to the burning sensation of "acid" indigestion, to more severe abdominal pain. Indigestion may also be accompanied by nausea, vomiting, belching, constipation, or diarrhea.
In most cases, you can treat yourself if you:

◆ Stop eating for several hours.
◆ Avoid stomach irritants like coffee, tea, smoking, alcohol, and aspirin. (Take aspirin, if you must, with water, an antacid, or food.)
◆ Experiment to see whether lying on your side, lying prone, standing, or walking helps.
◆ Remove panty hose, undo your belt, and loosen tight-fitting clothing.
◆ Avoid milk. It stimulates the stomach to produce more acid rather than relieving "acid" indigestion.

To prevent indigestion:

◆ Avoid foods that upset your stomach.
◆ Do not overeat.
◆ Try to avoid erratic habits such as missing sleep, eating at irregular times, and going on bizarre diets.
◆ Before a long car trip, eat only a light meal or wait one or two hours after a heavy meal.

Call a doctor immediately if indigestion is severe and accompanied by difficulty in breathing, sudden nausea or vomiting, fainting, rapid heartbeats, heavy sweating, or a cold, clammy feeling.

Infant Diarrhea While adults can tolerate diarrhea for several days before calling a doctor, the life of an infant under age two may quickly be threatened by dehydration from diarrhea. Thus, your baby should be taken to a doctor or a hospital immediately if:

♦ Stools suddenly turn loose or watery.

♦ Stools contain pus or blood.

♦ Fever rises to 101°F. or more.

♦ Vomiting occurs.

Keep older children with diarrhea in bed and administer fluids and soft foods.

Intestinal Gas   A petard, or expulsion of gas from the rectum, is far more threatening to social convention than to health. Still, if you want to cut down on your gas production:

♦ Eat bland or low-fat foods that are easy to digest.

♦ Avoid gas-generating or gas-containing foods like onions, garlic, beans, cabbage, cauliflower, broccoli, brussels sprouts, milk, milkshakes, meringue, soufflés, and carbonated beverages.

♦ Stop eating when you feel uncomfortable.

♦ Exercise daily. Walk whenever possible, climb stairs, jog, and avoid sitting for hours at a time.

♦ Remember that during times of stress, tension, or excitement, many people tend to swallow air, and this leads to flatulence.

♦ If you are an air swallower, correct the features that make it worse: ill-fitting dentures, nasal congestion, smoking, chewing gum, gasping, talking and eating too fast, and sipping through straws.

♦ If you already have gas pains, relieve them by rocking back and forth with your knees held close to your chest.

♦ Try lying prone over some pillows or standing on your head. The latter works because gas tends to rise.

♦ Or try a modified headstand and bend over the edge of a bed with your legs on the mattress and hands on the floor.

♦ A heating pad on your abdomen may also provide some relief.

♦ Gas sufferers often dose themselves with antacids, but

they do not work unless they contain simethicone, which disperses gas bubbles.

♦ Activated charcoal has not been proven effective against intestinal gas and, according to a Food and Drug Administration panel of experts, should not be taken for longer than seven days, at a dosage limited to ten grams daily.

♦ Bicarbonate of soda helps the intestine expel gas but should be used only temporarily in emergencies because it can contribute to high blood pressure and disturb body metabolism.

Irritable Bowel Syndrome Also known as spastic colon, irritable colon, nervous diarrhea, or functional bowel disease, this is the "common cold" of the digestive tract. Irritable bowel syndrome causes at least fifty percent of all digestive problems and is the one digestive disease for which doctors agree the underlying cause is emotional. It has been called the "intestinal equivalent of weeping."

Although no organic cause for irritable bowel syndrome can be found, it disrupts the functions and behavior of the colon, resulting in alternating attacks of diarrhea and constipation, cramping abdominal pain, and possibly gas pains, loss of appetite, frequent belching, heart palpitations, shortness of breath, and fatigue after mild exertion. These symptoms occur because the heart and lungs are stimulated by the same parts of the nervous system as the colon.

No one treatment works, but many measures help:

♦ Stop and think: are you under any kind of stress? If the answer is yes, you may feel better just from knowing the cause of your problem.

♦ Avoid fried and other foods that seem to make diarrhea worse.

♦ Avoid coffee, alcohol, and smoking.

♦ Eat slowly and chew food thoroughly.

♦ Drink plenty of fluids.

♦ Remember that fatigue or other illnesses such as flu can cause inflammatory bowel disease to flare up.

♦ Take Lomotil or belladonna to relieve occasional

cramps and diarrhea, but do not take these drugs regularly.

♦ Do not resort to laxatives for constipation. They irritate the colon and can lead to laxative abuse.

♦ Increase the fiber in your diet by eating whole bran, fruits, and vegetables, or try bulk laxatives such as Metamucil to relieve alternating diarrhea and constipation. Experiment to see what dose produces regular bowel movements.

If your condition does not respond to these measures, see a doctor. Some doctors prescribe bland diets, mild sedatives, smooth muscle relaxants, and antispasmodic drugs for more severe cases. There is no surgical treatment for irritable bowel syndrome.

Motion Sickness The classic symptoms of motion sickness include queasy stomach, heavy salivation, pallor, cold sweating, nausea, vomiting, indifference to social surroundings, depression, and a wish to be left alone and / or to die.

To avoid this terrible state:

♦ Rest up before a trip. Fatigue worsens motion sickness.

♦ Take frequent, short trips in a car to accustom yourself to driving.

♦ Jog or swim. These sports accustom your balance system to movement.

♦ Watch the distant scenery rather than the dashboard or nearby telephone poles whizzing by.

♦ At sea, remain on deck, gaze at the distant horizon, and keep busy.

♦ In the air, take a seat over the wheels because the tail moves more than the body of the plane.

♦ Avoid reading, tobacco smoke, and unpleasant odors. They may make motion sickness worse.

♦ Avoid eating or drinking for an hour before a trip and don't snack enroute.

♦ Remember, one drink might help, but more make motion sickness worse.

♦ Take motion sickness drugs twenty to sixty minutes

before departing, and remember that they may cause drowsiness.

A doctor must administer motion sickness drugs by injection once vomiting has started.

Nausea and Vomiting Nausea is that unpleasant urge to throw up. Vomiting occurs when the lower part of your stomach contracts violently and the pyloric, or "exit," valve to the small intestine remains firmly shut, forcing your stomach contents up and out.

Some people induce vomiting by taking syrup of ipecac or activated charcoal. The finger-down-the-throat method is also effective. You should not induce vomiting when someone has swallowed a strong acid or alkali or other corrosive substance such as kerosene, gasoline, cleaning fluids, lighter fluid, toilet-bowl cleaner, turpentine, ammonia, bleach, insect sprays, or liquid furniture polish.

To prevent vomiting:

♦ Eat smaller portions of food.
♦ Avoid drinking large quantities of fluids, especially at mealtimes, and take small sips.
♦ Loosen clothing and get some fresh air.
♦ Relax. Fatigue makes nausea and vomiting worse.

To recover from vomiting:

♦ Put nothing in your stomach for two to three hours after the last bout. Then try clear, cool beverages such as water, iced tea, or flat gingerale.
♦ If you tolerate these well, start solid foods two to three hours later.
♦ Starting with soups, Jell-O, applesauce, toast, and crackers, work up slowly to a normal diet.
♦ Suck on ice chips if nothing else will stay down.

If vomiting persists, see a doctor. One danger of vomiting, especially for children, is dehydration, which is more likely to occur if the child has diarrhea as well. See a doctor if a child under two loses all fluid intake for six hours, if a child between two and ten years old loses all fluid intake for eight to ten hours, or if an adult loses all fluid intake for twelve hours. And see a physician immediately if the vomitus appears black or bloody.

Pancreatitis Acute pancreatitis, an inflammation of the pancreas — the most powerful digestive organ in your body — is a medical emergency. It causes excruciating abdominal pains just above or around your navel, which may radiate to your back. The pain is made worse by moving or pressing on your abdomen, or by eating a meal. You may experience nausea and vomiting, constipation, jaundice, and rapid pulse rate. In very severe cases, you may go into shock.

Pancreatitis must be treated in the hospital, but once you recover, your doctor will determine whether gallstones or excessive alcohol consumption has caused the problem. Your doctor can remove gallstones, but if alcohol is the cause of your problem, you must stop drinking. To prevent further attacks, your doctor will probably recommend that you:

- Eat a low-fat diet.
- Limit food intake to frequent snacks.
- Reduce alcohol consumption to one drink a day or less.
A substantial percentage of alcoholics develop pancreatitis and will not give up their cocktails, even at the price of their lives.

Ulcerative Colitis People with ulcerative colitis have an inflammation of the inner lining of the large intestine. They may also have open sores in the colon, which cause pain that resembles abdominal cramps. They may have high fever, gas, and bloody diarrhea that occurs up to two dozen times a day and may last for weeks or years.

During an attack of ulcerative colitis, your doctor will probably recommend that you:

- Get plenty of bed rest.
- Eat a high-protein, high-fiber diet to replenish nutrients and control diarrhea.
- Replace fluids lost through diarrhea.
- Relieve abdominal cramps with an electric heating pad or hot-water bottle.

♦ Lie down after meals to reduce abdominal cramps and the number of bowel movements.

If an attack of ulcerative colitis is severe — involving high fever, significant bleeding from the rectum, abdominal distention, drowsiness, or severe pain — you may have a serious complication requiring immediate hospital care, intravenous feeding, antibiotics, and possibly surgery.

Ulcers The symptoms were described back in 350 B.C.: a steady, gnawing pain at the tip of the breastbone that may resemble heartburn, but is usually more severe and lasts longer. Frequently, ulcer pain occurs day after day at the same hour just *before* a meal, whereas heartburn occurs *after* a meal. Ulcer pain is usually relieved by eating, and then recurs thirty minutes to two hours later. Nocturnal pain between midnight and 2:00 A.M. is common because an empty stomach is more vulnerable to burning digestive acids that eat away eroded areas in the lining of the stomach. Sometimes ulcers cause no pain at all, and are discovered when they bleed and cause you suddenly to vomit a material that resembles coffee grounds, or to pass bloody or dark, tarry stools. If this happens, you will hardly need to be told: see a doctor immediately.

Most ulcer patients are advised to:

♦ Eat frequently during the day. What you eat is determined by you, your stomach, and your doctor.

♦ Avoid anything that damages your stomach or makes it produce more acid: cigarettes, aspirin, hard liquor, coffee, hot and spicy foods, and carbonated drinks containing caffeine.

♦ Remember that milk, once thought to relieve ulcers by neutralizing stomach juices, apparently soothes the mind more than the body. Recent studies show that its net effect is to *increase* stomach acidity, although it relieves ulcer pain for ten to fifteen minutes.

♦ If you crave caffeine, remember that one cup of tea contains about one-third the caffeine in one cup of coffee.

♦ Learn to handle stress and anger. If pressures are too

great, back off and give yourself a chance to say, "Whew!"

♦ Don't start the day with a cigarette and coffee for breakfast, especially not the day you're scheduled for a stressful meeting with your boss.

♦ Don't take a "quick drink" of liquor on an empty stomach to calm your nerves.

♦ Take medications as prescribed by your doctor and don't stop just because symptoms go away. It usually takes six weeks to cure an ulcer, even though symptoms disappear in a few days.

♦ Antacids remain the classic treatment for ulcers because they neutralize stomach secretions. Take them one to three hours after meals, at bedtime, and any other time you feel ulcer pain.

♦ Some antacids like Maalox and Gelusil are more effective because they are not absorbed through the stomach walls and do not stimulate the stomach to secrete even more acid.

♦ Liquid antacids work better than tablets, which must be chewed thoroughly to effectively coat your stomach lining.

♦ The medication physicians most often prescribe for ulcers is cimetidine, a new drug that relieves and heals ulcers, and apparently keeps them healed.

Evaluating Your Physician

An important part of health and self-care is to have a physician in whom you have confidence. To evaluate your present physician or to find a new one, ask yourself these questions:

♦ Do you and your doctor trust one another?

♦ Does your doctor listen to you and answer all your questions, or is your doctor vague, impatient, and unwilling to explain the nature and treatment of your illness? *If so, find another doctor.*

♦ Does your doctor take a thorough "history" and ask about drugs you are taking, as well as about your physical and emotional problems?

◆ Does your physician automatically prescribe drugs rather than explore the real causes of your health problem?

◆ Does your doctor return phone calls, give you emergency appointments, and provide a colleague to take care of you during his or her absence?

◆ Does your doctor pressure you to have surgery and discourage you from seeking a second opinion about surgery or major diagnostic tests? *If so, change doctors.*

Remember that you are paying for your doctor's services and entrusting him or her with your life and health. But remember, too, that you owe your doctor cooperation, honesty, and full effort to maintain a contract of equals. Sometimes this means recognizing that the medical profession, for all its achievements, can do only a certain amount to keep your body and digestion running well. You, not your doctor, bear ultimate responsibility for your health. This means you must:

◆ Understand your digestive system and what can go wrong with it.

◆ Make healthful changes in your lifestyle and diet.

◆ Remember that emotional self-care may be the most important kind of care, since digestive diseases are so clearly identified with the stresses of modern living.

APPENDIXES
INDEX

APPENDIX A

Helping Hands

National Digestive Diseases Education and Information Clearinghouse
1555 Wilson Boulevard, Suite 600
Rosslyn, Virginia 22209
(301) 496-9707

This is an information service of the National Institute of Arthritis, Diabetes, and Digestive and Kidney Diseases. The Clearinghouse coordinates a national effort to educate the public, patients, their families, physicians, and other health care providers about the prevention and management of digestive diseases. The Clearinghouse provided the following list of lay and professional organizations concerned with digestive diseases:

Lay

American Celiac Society (ACS)
45 Gifford Avenue
Jersey City, New Jersey 07304
(201) 432-1207

ACS provides information on how to follow a gluten-free diet; helps members locate gluten-free specialty foods; and encourages retailers to make such products available. ACS also conducts research and provides educational programs and publications.

245

American Cancer Society (ACS)
777 Third Avenue
New York, New York 10017
(212) 371-2900

The ACS is a voluntary organization dedicated to the control and eradication of cancer. The Society includes more than two million volunteers who help educate the public to the dangers of cancer and the possibilities of cure, educate the medical profession to the latest advances in the diagnosis and treatment of cancer, provide direct service to cancer patients and their families, and support the Society's huge research program.

American Digestive Disease Society (ADDS)
7720 Wisconsin Avenue
Bethesda, Maryland 20814
(301) 652-5524

ADDS distributes materials on digestive diseases to its members and the general public, including information about specific functional disorders, diagnosis and treatment, nutrition and diet, emotional and psychological difficulties and their relation to health, and research findings and advanced treatment techniques. ADDS sponsors *Gutline*, a telephone call-in service that provides counseling by gastroenterologists and other health professionals. The society has also developed dietary plans for people with digestive problems.

American Hepatic Foundation (AHF)
P. O. Box 1005
Williamston, North Carolina 27892
(919) 792-5279

The AHF provides support for research and education on the causes, diagnosis, prevention, and treatment of liver diseases. It sponsors competitions and gives awards.

American Liver Foundation (ALF)
30 Sunrise Terrace
Cedar Grove, New Jersey 07009
(201) 857-2626

The ALF's purpose is to improve the understanding and prevention of liver diseases and to find cures for liver diseases through professional, patient, and public education, and support of the research training of young investigators. The ALF provides a referral service, a communications network through its publications *Progress* and *Sharing Hopes and Cares*, and support groups through its chapters.

Center for Ulcer Research and Education (CURE) Foundation
11661 San Vincente Boulevard, Suite 304
Los Angeles, California 90049
(312) 825-5091

CURE funds and conducts research on the cause, cure, and prevention of peptic ulcer disease. It sponsors conferences and symposia on research developments and publishes educational materials.

Children's Liver Foundation (CLF)
28 Highland Avenue
Maplewood, New Jersey 07040
(201) 761-1111

The goals of the CLF are to set up a support system for parents of afflicted children, raise funds for liver research, and educate the public and health professionals about liver disease in children. The CLF awards research grants, conducts symposia, and distributes educational brochures.

Cystic Fibrosis Foundation (CF Foundation)
6000 Executive Boulevard, Suite 309
Rockville, Maryland 20852
(301) 881-9130

The Foundation supports cystic fibrosis-related research and training through grants and fellowships. It supports 127 cystic fibrosis medical centers, publishes educational materials, and maintains a database of patient information for use by researchers and other scientists.

Dean Thiel Foundation (DTF)
30 Sunrise Terrace
Cedar Grove, New Jersey 07009
(201) 857-2626

The DTF encourages young scientific investigators to enter the field of liver research by supporting research fellowships. It disseminates literature and assists patients and parents of children with liver disease through a communications network and through mutual help groups. The DTF is an affiliate of the American Liver Foundation.

The Gail I. Zuckerman Foundation
2600 Netherland Avenue
Riverdale, New York 10463
(212) 884-7950

The Foundation was established in 1967. Its primary function is to raise funds for research in the chronic liver diseases of children. Support is provided for basic research programs and fellowships. The Foundation has been actively involved with research programs since its inception.

The Gastro-Intestinal Research Foundation (GIRF)
Six North Michigan Avenue, Suite 1318
Chicago, Illinois 60602
(312) 332-1350

The GIRF was founded in 1962 to help combat gastrointestinal disorders. GIRF has supported research and training programs at the Center for the Study of Digestive Diseases by raising annual operating support and emergency funds. GIRF has also made interim financing available for appointments to the staff and supported the advanced training of young scientists.

Gluten Intolerance Group (GIG)
26604 Dover Court
Kent, Washington 98031
(206) 854-9606

In existence for over six years, GIG provides educational materials and emotional support to over six hundred members. Other services include counseling for persons with celiac sprue and their families, educational seminars for health professionals, and a telephone "hot line" for immediate information and referral. GIG also supplies hard-to-get, gluten-free ingredients and products to its membership.

Lifeline Foundation, Inc.
Two Osprey Road
Sharon, Massachusetts 02067
(617) 784-3250

The Lifeline Foundation represents those who are fed parenterally and enterally, including victims of digestive diseases such as Crohn's disease, trauma and cancer patients, and infants with birth defects. The group offers patient support through a call-in service, a newsletter, and conferences where lifeliners share information and techniques. The Foundation also informs the public, health care professionals, the health care industry, and public officials of the special problems of lifeliners.

National Association of Anorexia Nervosa and Eating Disorders, Inc.
Box 271
Highland Park, Illinois 60035

This organization is dedicated to alleviating the problems of eating disorders by assisting in the development of self-help groups for anorectics and their families, helping those seeking referrals for therapy, finding and providing in-depth information about specialties and treatment techniques of various therapists and treatment centers, encouraging research, and promoting programs for early detection of anorexia nervosa through educational programs for schools, families, health professionals, and the general public.

National Foundation for Ileitis and Colitis (NFIC)
295 Madison Avenue
New York, New York 10017
(212) 685-3440

The NFIC supports both basic and clinical research through grants and awards and also produces literature and public service programs to educate the public about inflammatory bowel disease. It instructs health care professionals in the diagnosis and treatment of these diseases through medical seminars, publications, and exhibits at medical conventions.

Pediatric Liver Research Foundation (PLRF)
113 Pacific Avenue
Collingswood, New Jersey 08108
(609) 854-1510

The PLRF supports research fellowships in pediatric liver diseases; disseminates information to the public through media, literature, and educational meetings; and coordinates mutual help groups for parents of children with liver disease. The PLRF is an affiliate of the American Liver Foundation.

United Ostomy Association (UOA)
2001 West Beverly Boulevard
Los Angeles, California 90057
(213) 413-5510

UOA stresses adjustment to living with an ostomy. Trained members visit ostomy patients to offer moral support and practical assistance. UOA publications describe ostomy care and management, anatomy, and sexual aspects of living with an ostomy.

Professional

American Association for the Study of Liver Diseases (AASLD)
Nuclear Medicine Service VA Hospital
First Avenue at East 24th Street
New York, New York 10010
(212) 686-7500

AASLD promotes the exchange of scientific information among physicians interested in liver disease and hepatic research. It conducts symposia and educational courses to improve the quality of patient care.

American Board of Pediatrics (ABP)
NCNB Plaza, Suite 402
1436 East Rosemary Street
Chapel Hill, North Carolina 27514
(919) 929-0461

A certification board, the ABP establishes qualifications, conducts examinations, and certifies those whom the board finds qualified to practice pediatrics as a specialty.

American College of Gastroenterology (ACG)
299 Broadway
New York, New York 10007
(212) 227-7590

ACG is a professional society of physicians and surgeons specializing in diseases and disorders of the gastrointestinal tract and accessory organs of digestion, including those of nutrition.

American College of Radiology (ACR)
20 N. Wacker Drive
Chicago, Illinois 60606
(312) 236-4963

The ACR is a professional society of medical doctors specializing in the use of radium, X ray, other radioactive substances, and ultrasound in the diagnosis and treatment of disease. Membership also includes physicists certified by the American Board of Radiology.

American Gastroenterological Association (AGA)
6900 Grove Road
Thorofare, New Jersey 08086
(609) 848-1000

The AGA fosters the development and application of gastroenterology by providing leadership and aid in all aspects of the field, including patient care, research, teaching, continuing education, and scientific communication.

American Hospital Association (AHA)
840 North Lake Shore Drive
Chicago, Illinois 60611
(312) 280-6000

AHA promotes better hospital services for the public. One division, the Center for Health Promotion, serves as a clearinghouse for information on hospital-sponsored health promotion activities. Center staff work in three major content areas: patient education, community health education, and employee health education.

American Society of Colon and Rectal Surgeons (ASCRS)
615 Griswold, No. 516
Detroit, Michigan 48226
(313) 961-7880

The ASCRS is a professional society of physicians specializing in the diagnosis and treatment of diseases of the colon, rectum, and anus.

American Society for Gastrointestinal Endoscopy (ASGE)
Thirteen Elm Street, P.O. Box 1565
Manchester, Massachusetts 01944
(617) 927-8330

The ASGE's purpose is to further the knowledge of digestive diseases by endoscopic means. It gives the Schindler award annually to the person who has done the most for gastrointestinal endoscopy during the previous year.

American Society for Parenteral and Enteral Nutrition (A.S.P.E.N.)
1025 Vermont Avenue, N.W., Suite 810
Washington, D.C. 20005
(202) 638-5881

A.S.P.E.N. provides educational programs and materials on parenteral and enteral nutrition for health care professionals. It maintains a speakers bureau, a register of institutions offering training in clinical nutrition, an employment register, and a library of audiovisual and print materials.

International Association for Enterostomal Therapy, Inc.
505 North Tustin, Suite 219
Santa Ana, California 92705
(714) 972-1720

Objectives of the Association are to ensure comprehensive quality care to persons having ostomies and related conditions; define and evaluate standards for enterostomal practitioners, allied health professionals, and students; accredit educational programs; and promote scientific research and publications.

The North American Society for Pediatric Gastroenterology (NASPG)
69 Butler Street, S.E.
Atlanta, Georgia 30303

The NASPG is a professional society of physicians interested in those gastrointestinal and hepatobiliary disorders affecting children and adolescents. The Society focuses on improving the quality and quantity of teaching, research, and patient care.

Society for Surgery of the Alimentary Tract (SSAT)
Department of Surgery, Duke University Medical Center
Durham, North Carolina 27706
(919) 684-6437

SSAT promotes research in diseases of the alimentary tract and their treatments. It provides a forum for the presentation of such knowledge and edits, encourages, or sponsors pertinent publications.

Society for Gastrointestinal Assistants, Inc. (SGA)
211 East 43rd Street
New York, New York 10017

The SGA is an organization of persons who work in the fields of gastroenterology and endoscopy with physicians and who staff gastrointestinal departments. Organized in 1974, the SGA seeks to promote the highest level of care for patients with digestive diseases and to maintain the highest standards of practice for gastrointestinal assistants.

APPENDIX B

Helpful Books

American Digestive Disease Society, *Living Healthy* (A monthly newsletter on various topics about digestive diseases, published by the American Digestive Disease Society, 7720 Wisconsin Avenue, Bethesda, MD 20814).

Brody, Jane, *Jane Brody's Nutrition Book* (N.Y.: Norton, 1981) (The best-selling lifetime guide to good eating for better health and weight control).

Deutsch, Ronald M., *The New Nuts Among the Berries* (Palo Alto, Calif.: Bull Publishing Co., 1977) (If you've ever wondered where American toilet taboos and hang-ups about eating and digestion come from, this book will amuse you in the telling).

Donleavy, J. P., *The Unexpurgated Code: A Complete Manual of Survival and Manners* (N.Y.: Delacorte Press, 1975) (Includes witty commentary on such social phenomena as farting and the proper outfitting of the well-appointed crapularium).

Galton, Lawrence, *Save Your Stomach* (N.Y.: Crown, 1977) (A carefully researched look at digestion, digestive diseases, and medicines people take for them).

Graedon, Joe, *The People's Pharmacy* (N.Y.: Avon Books, 1977) (A consumer's guide to prescription drugs, dangerous drug interactions, brand-name medications, and money-saving home remedies).

Kaplan, Marshall M., M.D., *Stomach Aches* (Wellesley, Mass.: Arandel Publishing Company, Inc., 1978) (One of the Tufts-New England Medical Center family health guides that briefly explains what you can do about various stomach problems).

Long, James W., M.D., *The Essential Guide to Prescription Drugs* (N.Y.: Harper and Row, 1977) (This book tells you what you need to know for safe drug use, and includes profiles of more than two hundred prescription drugs used widely in the United States and Canada).

Nugent, Nancy, *How To Get Along With Your Stomach* (Boston: Little, Brown, 1978) (A straightforward guide to prevention and treatment of stomach ailments, arranged anatomically and documented with an excellent bibliography).

Null, Gary and Steve, *Why Your Stomach Hurts* (N.Y.: Dodd, Mead & Co., 1979) (A serious book about serious digestive diseases, and some ways to treat them with stress-avoidance and diet).

Reyburn, Wallace, *Flushed with Pride: The Story of Thomas Crapper* (London: Macdonald and Co., 1969) (Story of the unsung hero who invented the flush toilet, complete with fascinating historical detail).

Selzer, Richard, *Mortal Lessons: Notes on the Art of Surgery* (N.Y.: Simon and Schuster, 1974) (The author's witty and provocative essays make the human body and its various parts — liver, belly and the like — the stuff of poetic prose).

Spock, Benjamin, M.D., *Baby and Child Care* (N.Y.: Pocketbooks, 1977) (The famous baby doctor imparts all the common sense you need to handle the stomach ailments of your child).

Tarnower, Herman, M.D., *The Complete Scarsdale Medical Diet* (N.Y.: Rawson, 1978) (Includes the allergy elimination diet and a healthful philosophy of eating).

Taylor, David M. and Maxine A. Rock, *Gut Reactions: How to Handle Stress and Your Stomach* (Philadelphia: W.B. Saunders Co., 1980) (When your doctor says your stomach troubles are all in your head, this is the book to read. Includes a very witty glossary).

Vickery, Donald M., M.D. and James F. Fries, M.D., *Take Care of Yourself: A Consumer's Guide to Medical Care* (Reading, Mass.: Addison-Wesley Publishing Co., 1976) (An enormously successful guide to help consumers take a more active role in self-care, find the right physician, choose the right hospital, and reduce medication costs. A section on digestive problems is included).

APPENDIX C

Guide to Fiber

DIETARY FIBER is the residue or remaining portion of certain foods — mainly whole-grain flour, cereals, vegetables, and fruits — which cannot be broken down by digestive juices, and which pass through the intestinal tract unaltered by digestion. Fiber, also known as "roughage," is a mixture of cellulose, hemicellulose, pectin, gum, and lignin. Cereals and other high-fiber foods add bulk to stools and enable their faster, smoother, and more regular passage through the large intestine. That is why a high-fiber diet both prevents and remedies constipation, hemorrhoids, and a variety of other digestive diseases caused or made worse by straining at stool.

The American diet consists mainly of highly refined foods from which the fibrous portion of the grain has been removed during processing. The average American consumes ten to thirty grams daily of dietary fiber, whereas the African villager — who eats a diet high in maize and suffers far fewer intestinal ailments than Americans generally do — eats about ninety grams of fiber daily.

Fiber is not an unmixed blessing, however. Diets high in bran can interfere with the absorption of iron, among other nutrients, although iron deficiency can be offset by getting enough vitamin C in your diet or by taking iron supplements. And high-fiber diets can cause gas and bloating, especially when you first switch to fiber. The solution is to alter your diet gradually until your body and bowel movements adapt comfortably to the change. Check with your doctor before changing to a high-fiber diet if you are over sixty-five, have bowel or kidney disease, diabetes, or other serious health problems.

◇   ◇   ◇

The foods listed below contain various grams of dietary fiber per one hundred grams of food. Cooking does not substantially alter their fiber content, although pureeing or mashing these foods will affect it somewhat. When you increase your dietary fiber, drink at least eight glasses of water a day, for fiber cannot act as a sponge and add bulk to the stool without it. Eat slowly and chew well so that fiber can absorb liquid and give you a sense of fullness. And eat a variety of high-fiber foods, gradually increasing your intake to forty grams of dietary fiber daily.

High-Fiber Foods	Grams of Dietary Fiber Per 100 Grams of Food	High-Fiber Foods	Grams of Dietary Fiber Per 100 Grams of Food
Bran flour	44.0	Parsnips (raw)	4.9
All-bran cereal	26.7	Sweet corn (cooked)	4.7
Puffed wheat	15.4	Rice Krispies	4.5
Shredded wheat	12.3	Broccoli tops (boiled)	4.1
Potato chips	11.9	Lentils (cooked)	4.0
Cornflakes	11.0	Carrots (young, boiled or raw)	3.7
Whole-meal flour	9.5	Spinach	3.6
Peanuts	9.3	French fries	3.2
Whole-meal bread	8.5	White flour	3.2
Brown flour	7.9	Celery (raw)	3.0
Peas (canned)	7.9	Summer squash (raw)	3.0
Peas (frozen)	7.8	White bread	2.7
Brazil nuts	7.7	Celery (cooked)	2.4
Peanut butter	7.6	Green beans	2.4
Baked beans	7.3	Peaches (flesh and skin)	2.3
Grape-Nuts	7.0		
Sugar Puffs	6.1		
Sweet corn (canned)	5.7		
Special K	5.5		
B.own bread	5.1		

High-Fiber Foods	Grams of Dietary Fiber Per 100 Grams of Food	High-Fiber Foods	Grams of Dietary Fiber Per 100 Grams of Food
Cabbage	2.2	Cauliflower (raw)	1.8
Summer squash (cooked)	2.2	Bananas	1.8
Turnips (raw)	2.2	Lettuce (raw)	1.5
Strawberries (raw)	2.1	Cucumber	1.5
Onions (raw)	2.1	Apples (flesh only)	1.4
Beets (cooked)	2.1	Tomato (fresh)	1.4
Carrots (cooked)	2.1	Grapefruit	1.3
Kale (cooked)	2.0	Cauliflower (cooked)	1.2

Other foods that are high in fiber include nuts, berries, dried fruits, popcorn, sunflower seeds, raisins, and garbanzos.

Index

259